T0250394

Extending Primary Care

polyclinics
resource centres
hospitals-at-home

Edited by **Pat Gordon**
and **Janet Hadley**

Foreword by **Barbara Stocking**
Regional Director
Anglia & Oxford Regional Health Authority

Series Editors **Pat Gordon** and **Diane Plamping**

Published in association with King's Fund, London

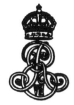

Radcliffe Medical Press

© 1996 Pat Gordon and Janet Hadley

Radcliffe Medical Press Ltd
18 Marcham Road, Abingdon, Oxon OX14 1AA, UK

Reprinted 1996
Reprinted 1997

British Library Cataloguing in Publication Data

A catalogue record for this book is available from the British Library.

ISBN 1 85775 029 2

Library of Congress Cataloging-in-Publication Data

Extending primary care: polyclinics, resource centres, hospitals-at-home/edited by Pat Gordon and Janet Hadley.
    p. cm.
    Includes bibliographical references and index.
    ISBN 1-85775-029-2
    1. Primary health care–Great Britain.   2. Community health services–
    Great Britain.   I. Gordon, Pat.   II. Hadley, Janet.
    RA395.G6E93   1996
    362.1′0941–dc20   95-47755
                                                                          CIP

Typeset by Marksbury Multimedia Ltd
Printed and bound in Great Britain

Contents

iii

Series introduction

Primary care development is arguably the most important topic for the NHS to get to grips with in the rapidly changing environment of the 1990s. This new series of books about primary care development is intended to be topical, useful and, before very long, out-of-date. It is based on the current work of the King's Fund Primary Care Group and the ideas, experience and inspiration of a number of people who have worked with us and shared their enthusiasms.

Primary care is often used to mean general practice. Here it is used in the broader sense to include the network of community-based health services which in the UK allow us to manage 90% of care outside hospitals; to manage earlier, safer discharge from hospitals, and to maintain people at home who do not want to be institutionalized.

From a position of relative neglect and invisibility, primary care has shot to the top of the NHS policy agenda. This has much to do with the NHS reforms and the drive to control public spending. Like all industrialized nations faced with ever-increasing costs in health care, we are experimenting with reorganization. Since hospitals use most NHS resources, this is where most attention is directed and primary care became the focus only as a potentially cheaper option. But the drive for efficiency and value for money coincides with other powerful influences which challenge us to examine alternatives to traditional ways of delivering services. If effective primary care really is the key to successful health services in the future, then recognizing its distinctive characteristics, and what we value about it as well as what we want to change becomes critical.

This new series is about ideas and services which are being developed and tested around the country. It is about work-in-progress in a period of extraordinary change. *Extending primary care: polyclinics, resource centres, hospitals-at-home* is the fourth title in the series. It discusses ways of extending the capacity of primary care to deliver the type of community-based services on which so much attention is now focused. Other titles in the series look at new ideas about the role of the practitioner, experiments in new kinds of primary care organizations, and new ways of managing practice-based primary care. We hope the ideas in these books contribute to the debate about the future shape of the NHS and are useful to the people working now in the middle of these major changes.

Pat Gordon
Diane Plamping
King's Fund
London

February 1996

List of contributors

Liz Adamson, Consultant Paediatrician and Medical Director, South Derbyshire Community Health Services NHS Trust

Jillian Alderwick, formerly Director of Primary Care, Birmingham FHSA

Franklin Apfel, Visiting Fellow, King's Fund, London

Egbert Bosma, Director, Institute for Quality and Applied Home Care Innovation (KITTZ), Groningen, Netherlands

Pearl Brown, Chief Executive, Riverside Community Health Care Trust, London

Pat Gordon, Director of Primary Care, King's Fund, London

Liz Haggard, Director of Health, Office of Public Management and formerly Chief Executive, South Derbyshire Community Health Services NHS Trust

Maggie Jee, Independent Consultant and Researcher in Health Care, London

Diane Plamping, Fellow in Primary Care, King's Fund, London

Julian Pratt, General Practitioner, Sheffield

Sarah Taylor, Consultant in Public Health Medicine, Birmingham Health Authority

Foreword

Fundamental changes in the Health Service demand a radical shift in approaches to patient care. The NHS is becoming increasingly led by the primary care sector. This has a greater meaning than simply more involvement of GPs in secondary care purchasing. It means that we start from where the patient is, in their own home and community. We provide care for them there and only move them into secondary services if and when it is appropriate to do so.

We need then to do a great deal more thinking and experimenting about what is appropriate in primary care. We need to develop the ability of those in primary care to deliver new services as well as helping them to develop their skills as decision makers in the use of and purchasing of secondary services.

This book is about developing and understanding primary care itself. It describes some current innovations – polyclinics, resource centres, hospitals-at-home. If developing primary care is to be about more than just relocating services from one place to another we need to be clear how these developments are different and whether they are cost-effective. Do they allow patients and carers to have a greater sense of control about what is happening to them; can we produce better patient outcomes by delivering care closer to patients; do we find in these experiments that we are extending the skills and capacity of the primary care team; and finally what does it cost?

These changes to shift care from the secondary setting to primary care have proved difficult to achieve. There are particular difficulties in our major cities and their outer rings. *Extending Primary Care* shows that it is possible to experiment beyond traditional boundaries in these areas. It will provide encouragement to people who work in these difficult settings by showing what can be done. With the new combined health authorities coming into effect in April 1996 this book could not be more timely as a resource for those who need to extend their understanding of primary care – in the fullest sense of the whole team of people in general practice and the associated community health services.

Barbara Stocking
Regional Director
Anglia & Oxford Regional Health Authority

January 1996

Acknowledgements

This book is based on a series of six King's Fund workshops on primary care development. Thanks are due to the participants and to the speakers who are listed below. Several of them have contributed case studies to this volume and I thank them for their patience and hope not to have caused offence with my alterations, omissions and interpretations. Janet Hadley wrote up the proceedings of the workshops which Andrew Harris, Jane Hughes and Julian Pratt helped to organize. Sue Lloyd-Evelyn and Madeleine Rooke-Ley kept track of the manuscripts and supported the work in countless ways. My thanks are due to them all and to my colleagues Martin Fischer, John Harries, Diane Plamping and Chris Shearin whose ideas enliven so much of our work in primary care.

Liz Adamson, Consultant Paediatrician and Medical Director, South Derbyshire Community Health Services NHS Trust

Jillian Alderwick, Director of Development and Review, Exeter and District Community Health Service NHS Trust, formerly Director of Primary Care (Assistant General Manager), Birmingham FHSA

Franklin Apfel, Visiting Fellow, King's Fund, London

Egbert Bosma, Director, Institute for Quality and Applied Home Care Innovation (KITTZ), Groningen, Netherlands

Pearl Brown, Chief Executive, Riverside Community Health Care Trust, London

Ashley Crumbley, Assistant Chief Environmental Health Officer, Liverpool City

Nancy Flannagan, Chair, Vauxhall Health Forum, Liverpool

Geoff Green, World Health Organization Adviser and formerly Coordinator of Liverpool Healthy City 2000

Marian Haben, Service Manager, Croydon Community Health Services Trust, London

Liz Haggard, Director of Health, Office of Public Management and formerly Chief Executive, South Derbyshire Community Health Services NHS Trust

Judy Hargadon, Chief Executive, Primary Care Support Force, North Thames Regional Health Authority, formerly Chief Executive, Croydon Community Health Trust

Maggie Jee, Independent Consultant and Researcher in Health Care, London

Tina McMullen, Health Visitor, Paxton Green Health Centre, London

Robert Marten, Practice Manager, Vauxhall Primary Health Care, Liverpool

Denis Pereira Gray, Professor, Institute of General Practice, University of Exeter

Sarah Taylor, Consultant in Public Health Medicine, Birmingham Health Authority

Kieran Sweeney, Research Fellow, Institute of General Practice, Exeter University

Christine Wall, Deputy Chief Executive, Liverpool Health Authority, formerly Chief Executive, Liverpool FHSA

Introduction

Assumptions about how we organize our health care system and about what determines our health are undergoing profound re-thinking. The current interest in a 'primary care-led NHS' and in 'effectiveness-based practice' is more than fashionable rhetoric. They are signs of a shift away from an unquestioning provision of 'inputs' to a questioning of outcomes, what works and how well it works, and appropriateness of care. Throughout the UK the reshaping of our health system is underway. In the language of the market, we have begun to re-engineer the supply side of the health system. In our major cities in particular the pressure is on to reconfigure hospitals and to find alternatives to traditional ways of providing services in hospital beds, outpatient departments and accident units. The challenge is to develop both the hospitals of the future and a primary care system capable of sustaining an extended role. This book is about some of the ideas and services that are being tested around the country in order to strengthen community-based health services and increase the scope of care provided outside hospitals.

From April 1996 the new health commissions (formed by the merger of district health authorities and family health services authorities) are in full legislative power. They are charged with implementing government commitment to a primary care-led NHS and a strategic shift from secondary to primary care. For many NHS managers this is a daunting prospect, not least because most make their careers in the hospital sector. This is likely to change as our notions of health care change to acknowledge the growing numbers of people whose needs go beyond organizational and professional boundaries. What takes place inside a hospital is significantly affected by what happens outside the hospital, notably in primary and community care and in housing. If we are to move in the direction of the strategic shift the government has espoused, we will have to build a better understanding of the NHS as a whole system rather than a collection of separate sectors. One way of contributing to this is to share our understanding of the characteristics of the UK primary care system and what we value about it, as well as what we might want to change. The chapters of this book are intended to be useful in this direction as well.

The NHS is a complex, social institution and as such we expect it to evolve and change. The current pressures for change, which affect all industrialized nations, include the following.

- Public attitudes are changing along with our demography. We are living longer and producing fewer children. We are also better informed and better educated than our grandparents and we want to be more involved in the treatment choices made on our behalf. Choice of treatment is much greater than it was and, for the most part, people want to be in hospital as little as possible.

- Disease patterns are changing in the industrialized nations. Chronic degenerative diseases have become a major cause of ill-health and their management over time has become as important as the treatment of acute episodes. Life expectancy has risen but with it has grown the tendency for disability to appear earlier in life. Institutions are not geared to managing chronic illness and policy initiatives are turning instead to an emphasis on prevention, user-centred services, and primary care.

- Advances in medical technology mean that less invasive and more effective technical procedures reduce the length of time patients need to stay in hospital, but may increase the time during which they need care at home. Many diagnostic, monitoring and treatment procedures which were previously only possible in hospital can now be carried out safely in or near patients' homes.

- Financial constraint, starting with the sharp economic downturn of the mid-1970s, has led to a policy emphasis on achieving control of public expenditure and getting value for money within the health system.

No one would disagree that health services should be efficient. It is the responsibility of those charged with delivering publicly funded services that these funds should be used to produce the maximum common good. As reducing public expenditure was the major driving force for the 1990 NHS reforms, the hospital sector which uses most of the NHS resources, remained the centre of attention. Primary care came into focus initially as a potentially cheaper option. But the drive for efficiency coincides with the other powerful influences which call for a re-examination of traditional ways of delivering services.

The desired strategic shift towards high quality, community-based services is unlikely to succeed without a well-developed network of primary care providers. In the UK, the two major providers of primary care are general practice and the community health services. Between them, they have the potential to deliver the policy agenda, but this will only succeed if their legitimate development needs are given due attention. What may be contained within primary care in Buckinghamshire, however, will not be the same as in Birmingham. Finding locally appropriate ways of resourcing primary care to undertake more or different services becomes a pressing managerial problem. Current government policy, however, is focused almost entirely on one aspect of general practice, that of the general practitioner as purchaser of services and the control mechanism for hospital referrals and costs.

Fundholding will probably contribute to the changing pattern of hospital services, and it will extend the GP's gatekeeping role. Practices (or groups of practices) with a registered population of 5000 can hold a budget for specific hospital care, drugs and community services. Practices with 3000 population can hold a budget for outpatient care and community services. There are 60 total purchasing pilot schemes now underway, in which practices can buy all types of NHS care. And any fundholding practice can join with others to share their management resources in the shape of a multifund. Fundholding provides a mechanism for general practice as an organization, rather than GPs as individual professionals, to engage with the rest of the system. But fundholding in itself is not a sufficient mechanism to develop effective primary care providers as the foundation of the whole system.

Each health care sector is becoming increasingly complex. We now differentiate between many kinds of hospital care – day surgery centres, trauma centres, community hospitals, tertiary hospitals, district general hospitals. Similarly we talk of primary care being extended. Despite the fears of some practitioners that this means nothing but a heroic extension of themselves, significant investment is now underway in new training e.g. nurse practitioners and community cardiologists, new equipment and new buildings to extend our capacity to provide more services in or near people's homes.

If primary and community health services are to be strengthened at the same time as hospital beds are reduced, primary care development programmes will have to pursue three strategic objectives simultaneously.

- Improving the basics. This means finding ways to make up the deficit and improve the quality and quantity of basic primary care, particularly in our major cities, to bring it into line with national standards. This means improving premises, re-training staff and resourcing general practice and community health services to provide the services required.

- Creating alternatives to family-based practice. This means adapting and extending primary care into more flexible ways of delivering services to meet the needs of the many groups of people, especially in cities, for whom the traditional family-based model is inappropriate.

- Shifting the balance in services from hospital to high quality, community-based care where this is clinically effective and appropriate. This could mean *containing services within* primary care which need not be 'taken over' by the hospital. It could mean *sharing services between* primary and secondary care. It could mean *transferring services from* secondary to primary care. In each case these shifts in the boundaries of care requires a shift in resources, knowledge and skills if the quality of services is to be improved.

The case studies in the following chapters can be seen as examples of development in each of these categories. In real life, of course, there is no such thing as a neat division of categories and the case studies make this clear. Resource centres, polyclinics and hospitals-at-home are examples of some of the experiments taking place around the country to extend primary care. They reflect the current concerns of participants in a series of King's Fund workshops on primary care development. All of them aim for a better fit between patients' needs and the resources available in different settings. One thing is obvious. Bricks and mortar are not enough. New buildings may be important in making up for deficiencies in primary care investment but without re-thinking the relational aspects of providing services, nothing of significance will change.

To put the case studies in context, chapter one discusses the distinctive characteristics of primary care in the UK, how it has developed and therefore how it might change in the future, and some faulty assumptions which hinder the search for shared understanding of what we want the total pattern of health care to look like.

Chapter two examines boundaries, or interfaces, which are central to the practice of primary care. They may change but they will not go away. Exactly where they are drawn depends on many factors including professional attitudes and practice, availability of equipment and resources, funding arrangements, and public opinion. Boundaries can be valuable because they can help individuals in complex organizations to gain a sense of identity and belonging. But boundaries cause problems when they block communication, create confusion, delay treatment, duplicate effort, cause people to undergo unnecessary treatment, increase costs, or reduce the likelihood of a positive outcome of care. Managing boundaries so that they do not become barriers is one of the major tasks of primary care management.

Chapter three looks at the development of a primary care resource centre in Birmingham to house a number of facilities which several GPs can use to offer their patients services they cannot provide from their own surgeries; and at the idea of a resource network or a 'resource centre without walls' in Croydon, which aims to achieve the same purpose without focusing on a building.

Chapter four considers alternatives to practice-based care and discusses the characteristics of polyclinics and urgent care centres, with examples from Eastern Europe and California, and a new service being pioneered in London to extend the range of care available outside hospital buildings.

Chapter five discusses two of the ways in which traditional hospital services can be shifted into high quality care in the home – Hospital-at-Home in South Derbyshire and the work of a Dutch development agency which is pioneering new forms of home-based care.

Pat Gordon
Janet Hadley

January 1996

Primary health care – its characteristics and potential

1

Pat Gordon and Diane Plamping

Introduction

Every developed country is showing a renewed interest in primary care, either as a means of controlling rising health costs or because its neglect is causing concern among users of the service. From being a minority interest a few short years ago, primary care has shot to the top of the NHS policy agenda and is now the focus of considerable managerial activity, not least in efforts to extend it. There is a problem however in the lack of shared understanding of what is meant by the term *primary care*. It is an abstract notion (though no more so than the terms *community care* or *secondary care*) and few professionals agree on a definition. For the most part, primary care is much less visible than hospital care partly because it takes place 'out there', away from the offices and institutions where most managers work. And yet one of the major planks of NHS policy in the 1990s is the creation of 'a primary care-led NHS' and a shift of resources and services from hospitals towards primary care.[1] If we are to move in this direction, we will have to build a better understanding of the NHS as a whole system, rather than a loose collection of separate service sectors which have grown from different roots and traditions, and to this day remain remarkably unaltered, despite waves of reorganization. Stereotypes persist. Creating a shared understanding of the words we use and the meanings we give them is one way of addressing them. In this chapter we examine the characteristics of primary care in the UK, its historical development as a clue to how it might change in the future, and some faulty assumptions which hinder the search for common meaning.

Characteristics

Primary care is not something which is done in one place or by one group of professionals. It includes rather than excludes. It can be described as a network of community-based health services that covers prevention of ill-health, treatment of acute and chronic illness, rehabilitation, support at home for patients who are frail or disabled, management of long-term ill-health, and terminal care. This network is linked in turn to a much wider social care network and this is what makes it possible in the UK to deal with 90% of patient contacts outside hospitals, to limit patients' length of stay in hospital and discharge them safely, and to maintain at home people who do not want to be institutionalized. In the NHS there are two main providers of primary care: general practice and community health services. Other providers are dentists, pharmacists and accident and emergency units, but the unique feature of our system is the combined potential of the two main providers. Recognizing their characteristics and what we value about them – as well as what we might want to change or to extend – becomes important. General practice brings one set of characteristics to primary care.

- It is delivered by highly trained **generalists** who can offer continuing and personal care for patients, described as 'biographical' care. This allows episodes of illness to be understood in the context of people's daily lives and helps in making the frequent adjustments which are needed to cope with chronic illness.

- It involves **teamwork** in which a growing number of professionals share aspects of patient care. Some of these are community-based specialists.

- It offers **first contact care** and is the patient's main point of entry to the health system (the other being the accident & emergency unit).

- It offers **accessible care** which includes geographical nearness, availability, language, culture, and old as well as new health problems. It is based on small organizations whose scale is critical to maintaining the non-institutional, personal care which many patients value.

- It offers **comprehensive care** which is not defined by sickness, age or gender. It includes disease prevention, health promotion, treatment of acute and chronic illness and rehabilitation. The availability of services 24 hours a day is essential to reduce inappropriate self-referral to other services.

- It offers **co-ordinated care**. The practitioner acts as advocate and information giver for her patient. This includes referral for specialist opinion and treatment.

- It has some responsibility for its **population**, 'the list'.

- It is activated by patient **choice**.

The community health services are provided by larger organizations through a range of both generalist and specialist staff. They bring another set of characteristics to primary care.

- **Support for general practice**. In small practices this can mean employing the district nurse and health visitor. In larger practices it can mean service level agreements for staff such as the community midwife or community psychiatric nurse.

- **Specialists in the community**. These include consultant paediatricians, stoma nurses, clinical psychologists, Macmillan nurses. Not every practice wants to employ a physiotherapist, for example, but the patients on every practice list want access to one when needed.

- Services for people with **continuing illness and disability**. This often requires skilful networking and liaison with voluntary and local authority agencies.

- Services which support **people discharged from hospital**. Some community trusts are beginning to carve out a vigorous home care agenda and their ability to offer safe, high quality nursing at home will determine much of the shift in services from hospital to primary care.

- **Services for well people**. This includes school health, child health, family planning, HIV counselling, health promotion.

- **Choice** for people without a GP or those for whom family-based practice may be inappropriate, for example, young adults seeking advice on sexual health, homeless people, or refugees. Community trusts have the flexibility to respond quickly to changing priorities and the organizational capacity to sponsor service developments. They are not bound by bricks and mortar.

- **Economies of scale**. Home loans and equipment are the obvious example which can only be provided efficiently for a large population. Economies of scale also support study leave and in-service training which may extend, for example, to include practice nurses developing their family planning or diabetic skills.

Community health services in the UK are as internationally unique, if less well known, as the family doctor services.[2] Their history is of professional and organizational development quite separate from general practice but, together, they form the building blocks which allow us to even contemplate the notion of a primary care-led health service. Between them they have the potential to deliver the NHS policy agenda of earlier, safer discharge from hospital, more frail people supported in their homes, better co-ordinated and more flexible community care, and more efficient and effective use of hospital resources.[3]

The new health agencies charged with implementing this agenda come into full legislative power in 1996. The functions of district health authorities (DHAs) and family health services authorities (FHSAs) have been merged and it seems likely that the new agencies will want to invest more in primary care, but not necessarily in 'more of the same'. In order to help put current events in context, the following section gives a brief analysis of how the UK model of primary care developed, and therefore how it might change in the future.

General practice development

The roots of general practice are distinct from those of both physicians and surgeons and can be traced back to the apothecaries of the 19th century (and earlier) who diagnosed conditions and recommended treatments, as well as preparing and dispensing medically prescribed therapies. In order to protect the public from 'quackery' in the rapidly changing world of Victorian Britain, the 1858 Medical Requisition Act was passed to help guarantee basic standards of medical qualification and practice. It also helped fuse three previously conflicting groups into one medical profession – the British Medical Association (BMA). Thereafter 'demarcation disputes between general practitioners and the more specialized physicians and surgeons were metamorphosed into medical etiquette'.[2]

In the early days of the NHS the emphasis was on access to health care for all. Two of the fundamental principles of the NHS were:

- to divorce health care from personal means, in other words to make access to medical services (and therefore it was hoped to preventive action) free

- to ensure that medical services were available to everyone, in other words comprehensiveness.[4]

This meant a new right to be included on a GP's list, but for many people this represented little more than an extension of 'the panel', though, importantly, it was an unstigmatized extension. Within a short space of time it was possible for almost the whole population to register with GPs. The really big change brought by the NHS, however, was access to specialist care in hospitals. The agreement reached between the Government and the British Medical Association left GPs as independent practitioners who continued on their pre-NHS path separated from the mainstream of NHS policy and finance which, in turn, paid little attention to the place of primary care in the health system.

Most managers probably know little about the first charter in the NHS, the Doctors' Charter but without understanding its significance and legacy, it is difficult to understand how our system of general practice has evolved.

During, the 1950s and 1960s an extraordinary movement developed within general practice. A remarkable cohort of GP leaders developed a theoretical basis for family medicine and a vision of how the role of a clinical generalist might develop within a national health service.[5,6,7] They created a Royal College of General Practitioners and a professional culture of audit and vocational training far ahead of the hospital sector. They challenged the notion of the GP as 'the poor relation' of the hospital specialist. Most remarkably they 'kept the faith' when most health care systems were turning away from the generalist to an increasing reliance on specialists. This is their gift to the current system which allows us to even contemplate a primary care-led future.[8] Other countries which lost their generalists, most notably the USA, face a 20-year development cycle to rebuild an adequate supply.[9]

By the mid-1960s there was growing awareness within the health service of the importance of the gatekeeping role of general practitioners and this combined with their professional leadership to produce the charter for general practice. This was a recognition of the need for public spending on general practice buildings, and for access to revenue for staff and equipment, and marked a significant shift in policy. General practice underwent a renaissance. The best undergraduates began to choose it as a career option. Departments of general practice sprang up in medical schools and further strengthened the theoretical and research base of the profession. Over the next twenty years the range and quality of services blossomed in many places. The new mechanisms were used to create models of care which are recognized as probably the best in the world.

However, it has to be remembered that this was a system built on professional development which insisted that independent practitioner status was necessary to safeguard clinical freedom; and which built up its collective strength and identity within a dispersed professional group by perpetuating a myth that all GPs are equal. In fact the developments were uneven and during this time the gap between the best and the worst probably widened. The good GPs took advantage of the terms of the charter but those who did not choose to, or who were denied opportunities to develop, fell further and further behind. By the 1980s there was an unacceptable degree of variation in general practice.

This was not the diversity which is entirely appropriate in small community-based organizations responding to local needs. Rather, it was a lack of accountability and a failure of inadequate mechanisms to bring standards to the level of the best.[10] The problems became most obvious in inner cities. In London in particular the Acheson Report painted an unremittingly bleak picture of uncoordinated primary care services struggling to keep pace with demands.[11] One of the legacies of the report has been persistent pessimism about the future of primary care in the capital, although measures were introduced which began to make the future look promising.[12]

However, general practice development at the top end of the scale had also begun to falter. The charter mechanisms contained some perverse incentives and even the good practices were pushing its capacities to the limit.[7] The cost rent scheme, for example, was no longer sufficient incentive to invest in premises when the price of property was rocketing. At this point, attention was deflected from the shortcomings of the system and turned instead to resist the market-led reforms of the Thatcher administration. The new GP contract was introduced and the long cycle of growing GP morale was ruptured.[13]

Firstly, whatever its rights and wrongs, the contract was imposed on GPs and completely undermined their sense of being in control of progress. Progress in primary care was intertwined with their own personal aspirations in a way which was entirely understandable given the personal commitment many of them had made to putting general practice on the map. They saw themselves as moving from being champions of primary care to being servants of the new FHSAs. They saw few additional rewards for good practice, but much additional bureaucracy. Other commentators saw the rewards for preventive care as progressive and supported the move towards some responsibility for the health of the whole practice population, as well as for individual patients.[7,14] Deprivation payments were also potentially beneficial but as they were not tied to performance, they too created perverse incentives. The drastic downturn in GP morale was not anticipated from what was seen as a relatively limited reorganization of general medical service regulations but, at a stroke, all the problems of general practice were laid at the door of the new contract.

The first waves of fundholding were built on ad hoc development by the same kind of practitioners who had grasped the opportunities of the 1966 charter. These are practices which are now able to operate as primary care organizations interacting with other organizations in the NHS. Fundholding has provided the opportunity for general practice as an organization, rather than general practitioners as individual partners, to engage with the rest of the system.[15] But fundholding is an insufficient mechanism to develop general practice. On the contrary, it seems likely that effective fundholding is dependent upon prior investment in practice development.

The current policy emphasis on fundholding concentrates on the role of GPs as purchasers of services and as the control mechanism for hospital referrals and costs. This will probably contribute to the changing pattern of hospital services, and it will extend the GP's gatekeeping role. But it is only one aspect of a health service which aspires to become primary care led. Just as important is to have well-developed primary care providers as the foundation of the whole system.

Community health services development

The community health services also moved a long way during the 1980s with the introduction of general management and their rescue from many years of neglect in the NHS policy world. Modern community health services are very diverse – some have grown out of hospital specialisms, others are closely related to social care. The range of professional staff is wide but nurses form the majority of the workforce (Box 1.1). Modern nursing in the community comprises a vast range of skills and specialist as well as generalist knowledge, but the inherited traditions of community nursing go back a long way and help to explain the way in which the community health services have developed.

Box 1.1: Community health professionals

Doctors
Paediatrician
Clinical medical officer
Geriatrician
Psychiatrist

Dentists
Community dentists

Professions allied to medicine
Occupational therapist
Chiropodist
Speech therapist
Physiotherapist
Psychologist
Dietitian
Audiologist
Orthoptist
Health promotion staff
Community pharmacist

Nurses
District
Health visitor
School
Community midwife
Community psychiatric
Community mental handicap
Macmillan
Marie Curie
Family planning
Stoma care
Continence advisor
Diabetic liaison
Discharge liaison
Clinic
TB
Nurse practitioner

Source: Audit Commission (1992) *Homeward Bound: A New Course for Community Health*. HMSO, London.

The roots of community nursing can be traced from the religious orders and charities of the middle ages through the poor law committees with their parish nurses to the reforming legislation of the late 19th and early 20th centuries, which established the basis for environmental health services between 1872–5, registered midwives in 1902, established a school health service in 1907, founded the College of Nursing in 1916, required home nursing for infectious disease in mothers and children in 1918, registered nurses in 1919 and reformed the professional body for home nurses into the Queen's Institute of District Nursing in 1925. When the poor law system ended in 1929 local authorities took over responsibility for community nursing.[2]

The NHS Act in 1946 introduced a tripartite structure which preserved the separation of general practice, hospitals and community nursing and allied services. The most immediate changes came about in the hospital sector. Building on wartime emergency experience; private, charitable and local authority hospitals were brought together for the first time to be managed under local and regional hospital committees. General practice was left to its own devices. Community health services were run by the local authorities but, with notable exceptions, the medical officers of health of the local authorities did little to develop them.[16] In the first major reorganization of the NHS in 1974, they were removed from local authority control and combined with hospitals under new area health authorities, where they became the poor relations of the hospitals.

From the mid-1970s, government policy began to give priority to developing 'community care'. Increasingly, emphasis was placed on the potential role of the community health services, but it was recognized that they suffered from managerial neglect and were not organized to cope with the demands likely to be placed upon them. By the early 1980s, however, the community health services had begun to establish an identity of their own.

Patients First was the policy document that led to this and introduced ideas of consumerism and decentralization: 'the closer decisions are taken to the local community and those who work directly with patients, the more likely it is that patients' needs will be their prime objective.[17] The policy directive that followed suggested organizing community health services into discrete units of management. The aim was to give them a single and authoritative voice. In the 1982 NHS reorganization, community units were created in most district health authorities, followed by the creation of general management at district and then at unit level. Many of these new general managers set about developing an explicit philosophy of community health service provision.[18]

On the nursing side they were aided by two influential enquiries established in 1985.[19,20] Both documented the uneven development of community nursing, which in some places was quite clearly 'in a rut'. Both articulated a vision of neighbour- hood nursing and primary care teams with skilled generalist nurses trained to assess local needs and provide individually tailored health care in or near people's homes. Changes began to be made at an unprecedented rate. With a responsibility to provide services to clearly defined populations, community services struggled to find ways of giving priority to disadvan- taged groups such as homeless families, housebound elderly people and minority ethnic groups.[21,22] Ambitious programmes of development were planned and, with a growing sense of purpose, came higher visibility.[23-27]

Policy makers at regional and national level, however, were slow to improve their understanding of the contribution of community services to the health care system. At the point where strategic decisions were being taken at the end of the 1980s, there was no clear idea of where the services were going or how they would relate to the other sectors. *Working for Patients* said a great deal about the directions hospital and family practitioner services should take, but nothing about community health services. The NHS was to be reformed by making hospitals self-governing and GPs more competitive.[28] In the field of community care – the 'other face' of the com- munity health services – there was just as much uncertainty. The Griffiths report recommended ways in which health and social services could work more effectively in practice to deliver government policy.[29] But the government's delay in responding to the report it had commissioned only added planning blight to confusion.[30]

In some perverse way, it seemed that just as the benefits of working for comprehensive, community-based health care were becoming tangible, community units found themselves vulner- able to fragmentation and the fear that the most 'marketable' elements would have to link with hospitals or entrepreneurial general practices and the 'non-essential' services would be allowed to wither.[3,31] The Audit Commission investigated[32] and confirmed that, like general practice, community health services were unevenly developed across the country. There was another enquiry into nursing in the community.[33] And, following the 1990 NHS and Community Care Act, there was surprise and incomprehension when some community units seized their opportunity and applied for trust status in the 'first wave' procedures of the NHS reforms.[34]

These procedures had been designed for hospitals and 'in as much as there had been any thinking about the whole system it had been neatly parcelled up between general practice and hospitals'.[35] However, this over-simple view has been challenged.[36,37,38] Some community trusts are now carving out a vigorous agenda for themselves and it is their capacity to deliver safe, high-quality care in or near the home that will determine much of the so-called 'substitution' agenda and the shift in services from hospital to community base. But in the uncertain environment of the 1990s where there may be opportunities for innovation and market positioning, there are still 'many assumptions, prejudices, and vested interests blocking or imposing change' for community trusts as providers of services.[39]

In the context of today's rapidly changing NHS, what is striking is the persistence of themes in community-based health care that have their origins in the development of modern practice well over a century ago. The dominance of hospitals, gender and invisibility are examples. Before the emergence of scientific medicine and the hospitals in which it is practised, home-based care was the norm and only the poor were cared for in hospitals. As this changed, community-based care waned and from the dominant medical perspective, it came to be seen as 'residual', to be provided after other care was delivered. Today policy thinking about extending primary care is still shaped by its relation to hospitals, as the case studies in the following chapters illustrate. Sorting out the claims of practice-based and community-based services and their impact on the use and costs of hospitals is likely to remain a major policy theme for some time to come.

The theme of gender is inescapable in a service where nurses are the dominant professional group. Nursing is 'women's work' which developed in its modern form over a century ago and still reflects its Victorian origins. Traditionally, nursing practice and its future direction have received scant attention from policy makers outside the profession. Since community nursing 'has always stood in the shadow' of hospital nursing and district nursing in particular 'has always existed outside the main thrust of nursing policy' it is hardly surprising if marginalization combined with gender to inhibit development in the community health services.[16]

One reason for the persistence of the 'invisibility' theme is that neither the social services world nor the health service has a consistent view of the community health services. There is still not a well articulated or widely shared view of its principle elements and its place in the continuum of care. Development may have been constrained precisely because the services have always been associated with much wider policy issues than illness, such as adequate housing or sanitation or telephone ownership.[40] Today there remains a widespread lack of appre-ciation of the complexity of delivering these services successfully and the diversity of agencies and professionals involved.

Some faulty assumptions

The third factor which would help in the search for a shared understanding of the term *primary care* is to challenge some faulty assumptions. One of these is that all GPs are equal – a GP is a GP is a GP. This is part of the mythology of the professional development model, discussed above, which has dominated general practice since the 1950s. In fact, there is widespread variation in general practice – some of it legitimate response to local needs and circumstances, but some of it unacceptable lack of standards and accountability. Agreement on core general practice standards and local contracts would help. Even a locally negotiated component of a national contract would be a step in the right direction for a community-based service responding to varying local needs.

Another faulty assumption is that *general practitioner* is synonymous with *general practice*. We often say GP, referring to a professional role, when we mean the practice as a provider of services, and vice versa. In modern general practice, the GP is one of a number of practitioners who work to provide the care for the practice population, the list. The NHS has an excellent track record on training, and nurturing professionals but is much weaker on 'growing' the kind of organizations to support service development.[41] In general practice, the incentives and levers for change are all directed through a contract with the individual (the practitioner) rather than the organization (the practice). Yet the reality of much contemporary general practice depends on the work of all the professionals within it and there are a number of experiments underway to find alternatives to the partnership as the only model for practice-based care.[42]

Another faulty assumption is that integrated patient care is achieved by including in one organization all the professionals who practise in or near people's homes. Community trusts have to manage many boundaries, both internal and external, in order to operate effectively. Similarly, because community trusts are bound by people and relationships rather than bricks and mortar, they have the potential for flexibility and rapid responses to changing local circumstances, but this does not come automatically. The gap between the best and the worst in the community health services is wide and their potential flexibility is often undermined by the tribalism common in professionally-dominated organizations.[32] They have the potential to increase the range of services to patients in their own homes which are qualitatively different from hospital outreach programmes. This will demand the development of equipment and specialist practitioners beyond the reach of most general practices. It will also place high value on liaison and boundary management with other agencies, both voluntary and statutory. Service level agreements and contracting and sub-contracting are likely to prove stronger linking mechanisms than exhortations to collaboration. Community trusts will have to find a way of managing the tensions and the connections between a general practice focus and a locality focus; between personal care and population care; between specialists and generalists, both nurses and doctors; and between community-based specialists and hospital-based specialists.

A health service guided by primary care?

'A primary care-led health service' is a fairly abstract notion. Sometimes the phrase is used to mean GPs purchasing hospital services. Sometimes it means relocating hospital services to a community base. Sometimes it means reclaiming from the hospital a service which need not be there. A more radical way of thinking puts a well-developed primary care system centre stage and emphasizes its core responsibility for providing appropriate services with the GP as first point of contact.[15,42] By getting this right, it confirms the place of primary care as the foundation for the appropriate use of the hospital sector and therefore, the effective management of its costs. In order to achieve the aim it has set itself, therefore, the NHS would have to concentrate on building strong primary care providers rather than focusing on only one aspect of primary care, the purchasing of other services.

At present, however, it is not at all clear who is responsible for developing primary care as new authorities are formed from district health authorities and family health services authorities. Nor is it clear that the hard-won experience of managers in primary care over the last decade is being recognized and extended throughout the new commissions, including board level. Without this, there is a real danger that mechanisms developed for the hospital sector will simply be recycled and almost certainly fail to deliver the desired outcomes. In order to succeed, a primary care development strategy would have to be built on four guiding principles which take account of its distinctive qualities:

- supporting the work of generalists, both doctors and nurses

- managing chronic illness as an emergent condition and not a series of events

- maintaining the scale appropriate to a personal care organization

- managing networks and boundaries as part of the core business.

:

Boundaries in primary health care

2

health care

Julian Pratt and Liz Adamson

Introduction

If a 'primary care-led health service' is to mean more than moving services from one site to another, it will require a comprehensive and consistent view of what we want the total pattern of health care to look like. Among other things, this means being explicit about the boundaries that exist between the three key sectors of our present system: primary care, hospitals, and community care. The 1990 NHS and Community Care Act which introduced the split between purchasers and providers of services and encouraged a plurality of providers, guaranteed that boundaries would multiply. Managing them so that they do not become barriers is therefore central to achieving high-quality patient care – and yet boundary management is not something to which the NHS has given priority. This is one of the key themes in the case studies in this book. They illustrate only too clearly that the range of stakeholders is wide; the cultures are different; arrangements for representation, consultation, and accountability are elaborate; and many of the ways of influencing action are subtle and indirect.

Many observers have pointed out the failure of effective working across boundaries in the health service and the interface problems within sectors and professions, as well as between them.[1,2,3,4] Hunter argues the need for effective boundary management in a health system which is becoming more fragmented, and describes the boundary skills that managers require, based on six roles identified by Donald Schon.[5,6]

1 *System negotiator* – the guide or middleman who serves as the vehicle by which others negotiate a difficult, isolated, rigid or fragmented system.

2 *Underground manager* – maintains and operates informal underground networks. May pursue goals that are functional but which have little or nothing to do with the formal policies of the agencies involved.

3 *Manoeuvrer* – operates on a project basis and is able, through personal networks, to persuade or coerce institutions or agencies to make the shifts required to realize a project that cuts across institutional agency lines.

4 *Broker* – makes deals, connects buyers and sellers, functions as a matchmaker at all levels of the organization.

5 *Network manager* – oversees official networks of activities, assuring information flows, referral processes, tracking and follow-up.

6 *Facilitator* – consultant, expediter, guide and connector. Functions at a higher meta level.

The authors of several of the case studies that follow describe the importance of these kinds of networking roles in their attempts to create new forms of partnership and joint working. Some clear commonalities emerge whether the boundaries are between general practice and hospital; community group and local authority; or generalist and specialist. These are explored further in this chapter by Julian Pratt and followed by Liz Adamson's case study of working at the boundary.

Understanding the boundaries

Julian Pratt

Boundaries, whether they be between individuals, groups or organizations, are frequently the site of failures of communication, understanding, cooperation and respect. Within a health care system, patients have many stories to tell of these failures. It is understandable that they should wish to find their way through the system without finding that its internal boundaries serve as barriers, causing confusion, delays, duplication, inefficiency and poor quality care. It is equally understandable that the system should wish to respond by offering to provide a 'seamless service'.

It is surely only appropriate, for example, that the advice given to the mother of a young baby should be consistent with the advice she was given during the antenatal period and her stay in the postnatal ward. The designer of a 'seamless service' might decide that this could be most effectively achieved if the midwife and health visitor were part of the same organization, sharing the same management. When the child goes to school the continuity of health education might be most effectively achieved if the school were another part of the same organization. This could also apply to the library service.

Do we want large organizations that try to do everything, or smaller ones that are good at what they do? Who would choose to wear seamless clothes, that just hang on the person, if the alternative is a well-tailored garment? The secret of tailoring is in the cut of the cloth (appropriate to the individual) and in the way the pieces are joined together (at their boundaries). The issue here is not one of market mechanisms compared with planning – in both centrally planned and private sector organizations there is a choice between autonomy for, or control of, the constituent parts. Autonomous organizations on a human scale foster identity, responsibility and a sense of belonging by both those working in, and those using, the service.

Primary health care is a much broader concept than the system of health care delivery. Emphasizing the partnership between health and other professionals and the community, it is built upon participation and intersectoral collaboration; that is to say on many organizations and their boundaries. Not only are there a range of organizations with specialist knowledge and expertise, but any society dependent on a complex knowledge and technology base requires both the depth of knowledge that is possessed by specialists and the breadth of understanding of the whole system that is possessed by generalists. The perspectives are held in balance at the boundary. Boundaries in primary health care may change, but they will not go away. They are central to its practice rather than some sort of mistake in the system design.

Several commonalities emerge from these boundaries. The first is the need to understand the nature of the boundary, which rests upon an understanding of individuals or organizations on each side of the boundary – not only of their structure, culture, vision, aims and policy options but also a genuine appreciation, valuing and respect for what each organization is contributing to the whole system. The second commonality are the connections across boundaries, in particular, systems of communication, systems of influence and flows of money. The third commonality is the powerful influence that can be held by individuals and organizations who identify their roles as working at the boundary and for whom the boundary is of central rather than peripheral importance – the 'boundroids'.

Understanding one's 'own' organization

For people to work effectively at the boundary of an organization they need to be self-aware and effective within the organization, in particular understanding who holds the power in each area of decision-making. They need to work with the formal and informal structures and within its culture. They will have to be in touch with the overall vision of the organization, both as a reference point and in order to be able to share the vision with other organizations. They also need to understand the aims of the organization as these will determine its desired policy options and thus the positions that may be adopted in negotiations with other organizations. Understanding at this level allows maximum flexibility. There are techniques available for expressing this understanding – an example of one of these, the 'Cultural Web',[7] (Figure 2.1), is given for a large general practice.[8]

An essential element of the organizational culture is how the organization feels about itself and how individuals feel about themselves within the organization. An individual's sense of self-worth and self-valuation in their professional role is central to their ability to function within an organization, and this is

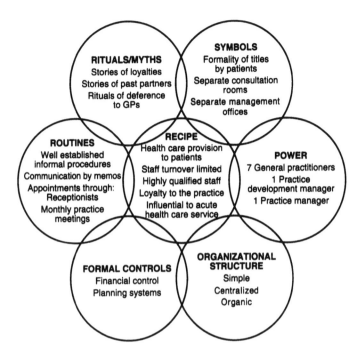

Figure 2.1: The Cultural Web.

particularly the case at a boundary where the individual may feel exposed. This sense of self-worth and self-confidence may be supported, or undermined, by the sense of safety and support for the individual provided by the organization. This involves clarity about the amount of discretion an individual has to make decisions, and the support given when they do so.

It is important to appreciate not only the strengths but also the limitations of one's own organization. This leads to an improved understanding of the needs that the organization has of others, and thus to better understanding at the boundary.

Understanding the 'other' organization

Working at a boundary requires an understanding of the 'other' organization as well as one's 'own' organization; and an understanding of the same factors are important – structure, culture, vision, aims, and policy options. Such an understanding may, even at the most basic level, be quite lacking – it is not unusual, for example, for a health visitor to find that her role, let alone the nature of her organization, is poorly understood by other members of her primary health care team.

A sense of respect for the 'other' is of particular importance. The generalist/specialist boundary, for example, is unsatisfactory if the generalist role is not understood, valued and respected by the specialist, and vice versa. Similarly, when one person is working within two teams, one of which does not appear to value the other, that person will have divided loyalties which may lead to considerable personal tensions, and impair the functioning of both teams and their working relationship with each other. Michael Balint described the relationship between doctor and patient, one of the important health care boundaries, as a 'mutual investment company'[9] – doctors and patients have the opportunity to build up considerable shared experience, which may include respect, that carries over from one consultation to another.

The sense of respect is particularly important when the aims of the two organizations are in conflict. In the NHS some (for example individual doctors and nurses) feel a central responsibility for the well-being of individual patients while others (for example, health commissions) feel a primary responsibility for the health of the population as a whole, whose will is expressed through parliament, ministers and the Treasury. Conflict between these two sets of values can be constructively handled if each understands and respects the aims of the other.

Knowledge of the boundary

The position of a boundary is usually the result of an historical process reflecting organizational and professional attitudes, availability of resources and public opinion. Boundaries will change and need to be re-negotiated over the course of time. There are choices to be made, which include not just the position of the boundary but its nature – in particular whether the boundary is rigid or 'fuzzy'.

To take a geographical example, an organization such as a community trust can describe the geographical area that it serves by drawing lines on a map (hard boundaries) or by specifying a central area of interest (with fuzzy boundaries). If community trusts have hard boundaries, patients registered with one general practice may be registered with a number of community trusts, making teamwork difficult. If community trusts have fuzzy boundaries they may, for example, accept the care of all patients registered with a particular general practice irrespective of the patient's home address.

Although boundaries do not need to be organizationally rigid, they do need to be individually clear. This is particularly important in the domain of responsibility – it must be clear who is responsible for following up an individual patient – generalist or specialist; it must be clear which community trust is responsible for the statutory visiting of an individual child.

Connections across the boundary

A prerequisite of effective working across a boundary is an understanding of the connections across that boundary, particularly the systems of communication, influence and finance.

Communication

Easy access and informal channels are frequently mentioned as factors that improve the understanding and respect one organization has for another. They can be enhanced by the physical environment at the boundary (for example shared offices, common rooms), but simply locating two organizations within one building is no guarantee of success.

Communication will frequently be about individual patients and the ways of best meeting their individual needs. It will also include the planning of service provision, and training. Sharing success is a powerful form of communication, particularly at boundaries, and can be an important factor in building motivation and increasing understanding and appreciation.

If an organization accepts that its boundaries are valuable it will ensure that communication across these boundaries is a central rather than peripheral aspect of its work. This means that, in addition to the easy access and informal communication, there will be regular opportunities for formal communication, for example, meetings which are part of the worker's job description and take place in paid work time.

Influence

Mechanisms for influencing the 'other' organization include:

- *Cooperation.* The most satisfactory form of influence across a boundary occurs when each recognizes a step that they can take which would not only meet their own aims but also those of the other. If a general practice wants to employ a nurse to provide more patient care and a health commission wants more clinical data from that practice, they might agree to share the costs of a nurse to do both. Cooperation is facilitated when each has past experience of cooperation by the other, and when the same people are likely to continue to work together.[10]

- *Compromise.* Each may slightly improve their position by co-operating even though not achieving their full aims.

- *Rational argument.* Where there appears to be outright disagreement it may be possible to reach a resolution by finding that there is common ground at the level of the aims or vision of the organizations.

- *Coalitions and alliances* with third party organizations which may be used to exert influence. These may work by increasing credibility (for example by commissioning an independent health survey from a university department) or by acquiring campaigning allies (for example by involving Friends of the Earth in air pollution measurements). Coalitions with the public are particularly powerful. A general practice may use such a coalition to persuade a local authority to make more resources available; a health commission can use a public alliance to overcome professional resistance to changing the culture of general practice in an area, by introducing a new general practice.

- *Threats and promises.* When none of the aforementioned is effective in producing change, one of the organizations may see a way of using threats or promises to shift the status quo.

Money

Understanding the financial structure and constraints of the two organizations is a first step in using the flow of money as a form of connection across a boundary. Transfers of money and resources can act as a counterbalance to transfers of work and responsibility. It might be possible to make better use of resources as a result of a change of practice (for example an increase in minor surgery in general practice), but if the costs are borne by that organization (as costs of time, equipment and supplies) while the benefits are felt elsewhere (more resources available in secondary care), the change in practice is unlikely to occur. Where two organizations are competing financially the boundary issues are likely to be determined by the financial competition, and areas of cooperation may be dependent on finding ways of avoiding this.

Working at the boundary

Strategies

Many improvements in working at the boundary seem to stem from the energy and inspiration of one individual or small group. One aspect of this energy is the ability to see 'threats' as 'opportunities', and to convince others of this vision. Another aspect is the willingness to take risks in enabling change. Probably the most important way for an organization to foster this energy and inspiration is to provide safety and support so that risks are not borne personally.

There are a number of common strategies that may improve working across the boundary:

- transitional funding

- asking the 'other' organization what they want

- working together (including permanent or temporary posts, secondments, shared posts)

- shared facilities

- joint planning

- joint training

- boundroids.

Individuals and organizations: the 'boundroids'

The strategies so far described have considerable potential to improve working at the boundary. Sometimes the most effective strategy is for people to have job descriptions that include the boundary as a major, or exclusive, area of work.

'Boundroids' may be informally-appointed individuals within one organization; they may be formally appointed by one or more organizations; or there may be a whole 'boundroid organization'. Some community trusts see themselves in this way. Not bound by institutions or bricks and mortar they can operate in a highly flexible manner between other more fixed parts of the system and lay great value on their adaptability and bridge-building capacity.[11,12]

An example of a boundroid, well established in this field, is a primary care facilitator.[13] The facilitator's work is to develop primary care providers and build relationships between general practice, community trusts and health commissions.

Boundroids need a mixture of skills that differs from those appropriate to working at the core of an organization. These include listening, facilitating, networking, building alliances and brokering. It can be an isolated position, between two cultures that may neither be in agreement nor share underlying values, viewed with mistrust from both sides. When the boundroid is successful, the two organizations may see the success as their own rather than acknowledge the part played by the boundroid.

Boundroids need to have a vision of their role, in particular its emphasis on process rather than attachment to specific outcomes that are outside their control, and a peer group to provide support.

Summary

Boundaries are an inevitable aspect of a health service tailored to the needs of its patients, and need to be actively managed rather than left to external forces and the accidents of history. They are an integral aspect of a wider primary health care approach, with its emphasis on participation and intersectoral collaboration. There are a number of common themes to effective working at a wide range of different boundaries.

- Understanding the nature of the organizations and their boundaries.

- Understanding and strengthening the connections across the boundary, particularly those of communication, systems of influence, and flows of money.

- Designating individuals or organizations to take the boundary as the centre, rather than periphery, of their work – the boundroids.

- Employing a number of specific strategies for improving work at the boundary, particularly by improving understanding and building trust and respect.

Working the boundaries – specialist service in the community

Liz Adamson

Boundaries are a permanent feature of the health service and working across a boundary, whether individual, intra-organizational or inter-organizational, will always be necessary. Professional practice and training has increasingly addressed the imperatives of managing professional–patient, professional–carer and professional–professional boundaries. The skills needed to manage these boundaries are being recognized and taught. The crucial areas of intra- and inter-organizational boundary working, however, are only now being considered. Professional and managerial effort to date has concentrated on removing boundaries rather than managing across them. The first step towards good boundary management is to recognize their permanency; they can be moved but they will not be removed. It is the duality of permanency with fluidity that makes the boundary area an exciting professional and managerial challenge which requires particular skills and attributes.

The specialist–generalist boundary

The professional inter-reactions between specialists and generalists illustrate many of the features of boundary working, and

27

the factors that disable or enable effective working across them. The specialist–generalist interface is one of the most common health service boundaries, and is often troublesome. Patients are probably more aware of this boundary than any other, a fact which itself implies problems. In an ideal world, patient awareness of professional and managerial interfaces would be minimal.

The NHS is built on the model of the generalist being the gatekeeper for specialist services, and this system requires transfer of information and practical arrangements to be made for a patient to receive appropriate care.

Although similar patterns occur at the generalist–specialist interface in other professions, the problems seem to be greater in medicine. Medicine is a demanding profession in terms of the expectations for authoritative decision-making and it is not uncommon for doctors to feel the need to erect protective personal and professional barriers. These are disabling factors for close boundary working. Enabling factors are: mutual respect for skills, a common knowledge base and a willingness to communicate and cooperate.

The generalist–specialist interface in medicine has been characterized, certainly until recently, by an assumption of superiority by the specialist. The greater in-depth knowledge of the specialist in the area of consultation and the vulnerability of the generalist to criticism inherent in the role of first-time contact creates this ambience.[14] From a patient's perspective, the process of crossing the boundary is formal, arcane and frustrating. From the professional angle, the main feature of the interaction has been mutual irritation.

The relative positions of the two professional groups are largely taken up during medical training, where radical change will be needed to improve relationships fundamentally for the future.

Medicine is taught by specialists within a hospital setting via a series of specialist modules. Generalism itself is taught as a 'specialist' module. This results in newly-qualified doctors with a limited range of specialist skills and little in the way of generalist skills. Those doctors who choose to specialize then move on to postgraduate training in their chosen areas without the opportunity to develop a broad common knowledge and experience base. There is evidence that the need for a more generalist focus in training is being recognized, but not necessarily explicitly, to enhance boundary working.[15] Some of the changes resulting from the introduction of GP fundholding suggest that progress does not have to wait for a radical change in medical training.

General practitioners with purchasing power have been able to change the attitude of specialists to one of increased responsiveness to their needs. It would be premature to conclude that this implies a sudden appreciation of respective skills but the improved communication is real and more cooperation and respect can be expected to follow. Forcing professionals into more overtly positive interactions may not be a fundamental solution to the problem but it can be a catalyst.

Another area that has improved, almost certainly as a result of audit, is the sharing of information between generalist and specialist. The preparation of management guidelines by specialists for conditions that cause concern to generalists, and the provision of information about rare conditions when these are diagnosed, are mostly very much appreciated by generalists. Specialists appreciate fuller patient details on referrals than they sometimes receive. The more direct contact there is between generalists and specialists the more likely it is that the value of this high quality information will be appreciated and mutually provided.

Technology can be expected to facilitate the sharing of increasingly high quality information but good boundary management must take into account the dangers of information overload and fatigue and the potential disadvantage of a reduction in opportunities for direct inter-professional contact.

Community paediatrics: an example of boundary working

Community paediatrics is a specialty which faces two ways. On the one hand it offers specialty services to general practitioners. On the other it sometimes requires the relatively high technology of the hospital paediatric service. The community paediatrician therefore acts sometimes as a specialist advising a generalist and sometimes as a generalist/specialist seeking greater specialist services.

Historically the specialty has evolved from an essentially primary care service into a distinct specialty.[16] This evolution has required the professionals to focus on the boundaries with general practice and hospital paediatrics in terms of both individual and inter-organizational relationships.

Elements of success

One important element in the evolution of the specialty has been its willingness to fill the gaps in services to children that were recognized as essential but did not sit comfortably within either general practice or hospital paediatrics. This has been crucial to the success of working with these other two professional groups and epitomizes one of the elements of success in boundary working. Two of the principle aims of a primary care-led health service are that specialist services should be driven by the generalist's needs and that services should be provided as close to the patient as is compatible with quality and effective use of resources. These principles can be adopted without professional defensiveness. In community paediatrics this has worked well at both the specialist–generalist and generalist–specialist interfaces.

Joint training

Shared training, both provided and received, has been another element in the success of boundary management in community paediatrics. Again, it has been a feature of both boundaries and it takes many forms. It develops the common knowledge base on which future interactions will be founded as well as providing a shared experience which contributes to individual and inter-organizational respect and communication; it is much easier to interact with another professional with whom one has a personal acquaintance and whose views and professional attitudes are known.

Joint posts

Joint hospital–community posts are becoming commonplace in paediatrics at all levels of training, as well as consultant level, and the individuals who occupy these posts are crucial to good boundary working. Having a commitment to, and an intimate knowledge of, both sides of a boundary, they can contribute enormously to the development of good inter-organizational working. Their dual commitment prevents organizational defensiveness and they frequently identify individual patient management problems that can be generalized to improve systems. With the appropriate skills they can effect real service improvements.

Joint facilities

The sharing of facilities has probably been more prevalent within community paediatrics than any other specialist field and has been seen as another element conducive to good boundary work. It would be over-simplistic to expect that working in the same buildings or sharing the same administrative staff will automatically result in better working relationships, but it certainly increases the opportunities for contact and for shared experience that helps communication.

Child development centres (see Box 2.1) have traditionally been places where professionals from different disciplines and different departments or organizations, work together in a variety of premises, also managed by different organizations, to provide services to children with special needs. In South Derbyshire the service is so closely intermeshed that, whilst offering at least a vision of a service planner's dream, it could easily constitute a contract manager's nightmare.

Joint planning

Probably the ultimate objective for boundary management is effective joint planning of services by separate organizations. Knowledge of boundary working is of particular importance as it would be hard to conceive of an organization that was functioning ineffectively if its boundaries were working well. The Paediatric Specialty Advisory Group (see Box 2.2) is a small medical lobby for paediatric services that is proving to have some value as a model of joint planning in South Derbyshire.

Joint management

Joint management has been seen as a means of removing boundaries and integrating community and hospital paediatrics. Joint management has been widely discussed and implemented in some areas, although generally in a limited way.[17,18] Where it has been implemented, it has not removed

---

Box 2.1: Child development centre

The main premises and administrative services are managed by an acute hospital trust. Consultant paediatricians from both acute and community trusts have registered patients and these patients might ultimately be seen by both acute and community consultants. Junior medical staff with acute, community or combined appointments train at the centre and have identical responsibilities. Nursing, therapy and some administrative staff cross the boundary in similar fashion.

Children are mainly seen at the centre but can also be seen in other health, educational and social settings within the district. In any of these settings, they may be seen by either acute or community staff.

Patients benefit from the wider network of services which result from this involved system. The potential disadvantage is confusion for both staff and users. This is not generally apparent, probably because of the joint training, monitoring and planning which is a feature of the centre and which results in the staff regarding themselves, certainly when working in the centre, as 'CDC' staff. They are certainly seen as that by the users who are not aware of the managerial complexities and hold the services in high regard.

The complexities of the system have required a degree of pragmatism on the part of business and contracts managers to avoid it foundering on a plethora of inter-organizational contracts.

---

the hospital/community boundary; in order to do so, huge managerial units would have to be created. What it has achieved is the transformation of some inter-organizational boundaries into intra-organizational ones. Again, the boundary has moved but this has not obviated the need for boundary management.

Joint management is possibly a sign of organizational commitment to boundary management but it would be naïve to assume that this commitment is always present in a jointly-managed service. It is certainly wrong to assume its absence in

---

Box 2.2: Paediatric Specialty Advisory Group

This is a sub-group of the multi-disciplinary Division of Child Health with a remit to lobby purchasers and to monitor providers. Membership is on the basis of care groups; children with acute illnesses, children with chronic illnesses, children with special needs, child surveillance and children with emotional and behavioural problems. This results in at least one consultant representative from each of the provider trusts. In addition, there are two general practitioner representatives.

The group initially met with many professionals involved with children's services and ascertained what the problems and difficulties were. These meetings alone were valuable in determining shared concerns, priorities and objectives and were thus a valuable communication exercise. The outcome was the production, as a first priority, of straightforward clinical management guidelines for a variety of conditions.

The group has also met with purchasers to produce a specification for child health services and continually deals with individual problems brought to its attention, frequently by professionals working at the boundaries. It is crucial that the individuals in the group have power to bring about change within their own organizations.

---

organizations managed separately. As a means of managing boundaries it is an option that clearly should be considered but only if it seems the most effective way of achieving the critical success factors identified above.

The boundary worker

Individuals who work at the boundaries between organizations should be recognized in terms of their crucial importance and particular skills. They must view evolutionary and, occasionally, radical change as an exciting challenge. Boundary workers must be effective communicators. They must be articulate in

---

their dealings with their own organization, and assertive but unaggressive, undefensive and non-judgemental in their dealings with other organizations. This communication and networking element should form part of their job description.

These attributes are additional to an individual's basic professional skills and need to be appropriately nurtured. It is essential that boundary work is seen as appropriate for senior staff with status and access to executive powers. It is inappropriate to assign junior staff with undeveloped interpersonal and negotiating skills and little power to an area of work that is of fundamental, though often under-recognized, importance to an organization.

Conclusion

The generalist–specialist medical boundary epitomizes the problems that can occur at boundaries. However, these can be alleviated by accepting the need for:

- specialisms to be driven by generalists
- services to be provided as close to the patient as possible
- greater respect for each other's skills
- enhanced common knowledge base
- improved communications across the boundary.

Community paediatrics demonstrates some of the practical ways that work focused on boundaries can be effective. In order to develop as a specialty it was necessary for community paediatricians to work with both general practitioners and hospital paediatricians to establish what services were required. The communication channels established have been vital in enabling the development of joint training, joint posts and joint planning. It is also important to recognize the time required for networking, both in terms of individual patients and of inter-agency working, the value of individual posts that focus on boundaries and of the professionals who fill them.

Factors for success include: skills of interpersonal and inter-organizational communication, seniority of professional grade and status and access to executive power.

Any organization that succeeds in ensuring that these factors are operating at its important boundaries is likely to reap rich rewards, not only in terms of its functioning at those boundaries, but throughout the entire organization.

Primary care resource centres – a means of supporting general practice?

3

Jillian Alderwick, Sarah Taylor and Maggie Jee

Introduction

General practitioners are primarily providers of health care for their patients. By and large, they want to deliver the best they can, and if they can't provide a service themselves, they want to obtain the best they can from elsewhere. Elsewhere may be a hospital or it may be some other 'centre of resources' which would enable the GP to offer more, or better services, or services closer to patients' homes. Currently one of the most popular ideas is to build or to refurbish a 'primary care resource centre' to house a number of facilities which several GPs can use to offer services which they are unable to provide from their own surgeries.

In this chapter, Jillian Alderwick and Sarah Taylor describe the origins and development of the Quinton Centre in Birmingham. Maggie Jee's case study offers another approach – a resource centre without walls. This is based on work in Croydon, South London, where three group practices came together with a community NHS trust to broaden the range of services GPs could access on behalf of their patients. This has more to do with the idea of a resource network than a resource centre, and immediately forces us to think about the issues of communication and inter-connectedness which are at the heart of good primary care services, whether they operate from one building or many. Both case studies highlight the complexity of delivering services at the primary level – multiple sources of funding, questions of ownership, relationships between professionals from different agencies – and the need for the skilled interface management discussed in the previous chapter.

Much contemporary general practice operates out of purpose-built, well-equipped premises where the GP works as part of a team of other practitioners to provide health care to the practice population. This includes preventive and anticipatory care as well as the treatment of disease and the management of chronic illness. But not all practices work like this, nor do patients want them to. Many general practices are small. They are human-scale organizations with domestic-scale architecture, which is an important part of their approachability. Patients like them but the services on offer are necessarily limited. In cities in particular there are many small practices which for a number of different reasons can be considered to be under-developed in today's terms. Imaginative health authorities have always looked for ways to support these practices. Providing buildings is one of them. This may be an entirely appropriate response to deficiencies arising from years of under-investment in the capital stock of primary care. Alternatively it may stem from an inappropriate transfer of hospital-based thinking.

A major capital development on a hospital site is complex and difficult but techniques have evolved to handle the issues. The nature of the complexity in a large primary care project is very different. Notably, there is no one systems organizer. In a hospital project, the hospital as a corporate entity 'owns' the development and usually has a single sponsor, such as the Region. In primary care there are often many owners and sponsors with one agency acting as broker. An FHSA, for example, could not own the property but could negotiate with GPs through the cost rent scheme to include general practice within the site. A community trust may own the site but have little leverage on the behaviour of neighbouring hospital providers. Are consultants willing to do outreach work from those specialties which meet the needs of primary care practitioners, for example? The regulations which apply to different agencies make joint financing a tortuous process. As the case studies show, the process of bringing many stakeholders to-gether is slow and time-consuming. Urgency is likely to under-mine success unless due care is given to the way services will connect with each other and relate to the rest of the system. They raise other questions too. What is the place of the private finance initiative in primary care capital development? Will developments with high start-up costs, such as resource centres, have the flexibility to adapt to changing patterns of use? Is major capital investment an appropriate way of developing services in primary care? Locating a number of services under one roof will not of itself produce better outcomes for patients, so will professional and organizational boundaries be managed in new ways? Will local communities participate in running local resource centres?

As yet there are few answers but the interest in building primary care resource centres continues to grow. A recent survey shows, for example, that the North West Region has em-barked on a systematic capital investment programme of some £20 million to create a network of resource centres throughout the region.[1] The survey reveals an enormous range of initiatives being developed under this heading all over England. These include:

• refurbishing and extending existing health centres

• developing polyclinics

• extending the role of community hospitals

• setting up nurse practitioner-staffed minor injury centres

• extending services offered by GP fundholders, especially hospital outreach clinics

• linking with local authorities to develop 'one-stop shop' information centres.

Each of these investments is likely to be specially tailored to local needs. They may aim to extend services in a number of ways by:

extending the capacity of local GPs to provide services to an accepted standard e.g. sufficient space for a practice team *extending* the ability of local GPs to work together to share resources or commission services

extending the access of the practice team to a wider network of community-based services e.g. clinical psychologists, nurse specialists

extending the access of GPs to specialist resources e.g. diagnostic services

extending access to primary care for those who find family-based practice inappropriate e.g. commuters, students, homeless people

extending local availability of hospital services e.g. outreach consultant clinic.

In chapter four we consider some of these initiatives under the heading of extending primary care by creating alternatives to general practice. In this chapter the focus is on resourcing general practice to enable more or better services to be offered to patients in a primary care setting. The aim is to get a better fit between patients' needs and the skills and resources available in different settings.

The development of a primary care resource centre in Birmingham

Jillian Alderwick

The Quinton Project refers to the development of a new and substantial two-storey building best described as a primary care resource centre but, locally, rather stuck with its earlier working title of 'local care facility'. Its purpose is to enable up to eleven local general practices to provide a broader range of services to their patients, including a number of services which would previously only have been available on a hospital site.

The background to the Quinton Project will be familiar across the country. However, some details of the background and certain aspects of the planning process are quite likely to prove crucial to the success of the project in the long term and are outlined here for more careful analysis. In January 1992, Birmingham Family Health Service Authority began work with a broad range of other organizations to develop a primary health care strategy for the city. The sheer size of Birmingham – with more than 260 general practices – means that there are examples of both the best and the worst practitioners and buildings. Regrettably also, the inverse care law is alive and well and living in Birmingham, with those whose needs are greatest often having access to relatively poor services.

In 1992 the wholly hospital-focused, and now discredited, plans for 'Building a Healthy Birmingham' were still blu-tacked on many walls – albeit a little dog-eared; but there had been no attempt to review the capacity of primary health care services in the city to grow and develop.

More recently, the need to substantially reduce hospital provision in the city has placed an unavoidable responsibility on all those concerned with health services in Birmingham, to ensure that any service which can be delivered effectively in a community setting is made available there and that general practice develops, not just as a 'gateway' to the hospitals, but as a core provider itself.

Better facilities

Two main themes emerged from the primary health care strategy – more effective use of resources and the shift of clinical services from secondary to primary settings. The strategy had several components including work undertaken to establish primary health care needs in different parts of the city and the scope for movement in a range of clinical specialties. GPs' views across the whole city were canvassed by an outside consultant who analysed their readiness for change and strategic develop-ment. In addition, a specific recommendation for Birmingham was that there should be a new programme for securing more effective facilities for general practice and community health services. In particular, it was recommended that a pilot project should establish a base for some extended primary care services which could not be realistically or economically housed in small practices. Also, importantly, this base should be seen as a resource to facilitate the shift of selected services from a secondary to a primary care setting. The working group which came together to explore this recommendation began a process which resulted in the 'Quinton Project', but it was by no means a group made up solely of commissioners. The working group comprised representatives of the FHSA, the Local Medical Committee, the Community Health Council, the DHA Purchasing team and the Department of Public Health, managers from both the acute and community units and two, sometimes three, interested and influential hospital consultants.

Some members of the working group were delegated and others had expressed a particular interest. Some knew each other well and others not all. 'Cultural differences' were apparent and there was generally a healthy scepticism about the nature of the project and especially its chances of ever being funded. At the outset and for much of the planning period the FHSA believed that the DHA had the money and the DHA believed the FHSA had it. Ultimately funding arrived unexpectedly from the Regional Health Authority (RHA). There was a strong political need to show something solid on the primary care side of the scales to balance the 'downsizing', of the Birmingham hospitals and when the RHA picked up the bill the opportunities for serious evaluation became much more limited.

Gradually, however, the commitment to placing more services in the community grew. It must be said that medical colleagues needed the most convincing and searched for a compelling rationale which, of course, did not really exist. Like many others, the team in Birmingham was working on an act of faith represented by 'extended primary care' and under tremendous pressure to build *something*. Over time, however, their resistance – if not their anxieties – diminished and there was a willingness to proceed on the basis that this was an experiment. As the implications of this were accepted the impetus seemed to come increasingly from the medical members and the provider managers. Sadly, the purchasers were relatively slow to give their commitment and to appreciate the workload implications for themselves. In a sense this resulted in, and continues to require, 'backfilling' purchasing decisions to deliver the vision which began to emerge.

As commitment to the principles grew, so did the enthusiasm of the group and a search began to identify a suitable site for a new building which could house some relocated hospital services and better facilities for GPs to deliver 'enhanced' primary care.

Finding a site

A site needed to be found in an area where existing GP premises were overcrowded or in other ways judged to be inadequate. A premises audit was designed and systematically carried out to ensure objectivity in this regard. It was felt that a minimum of approximately ten GPs was necessary within a one mile radius of the proposed site in order to ensure a critical mass of local activity and to offer the potential for bringing GPs into closer working relationships. This was regarded as particularly important by the FHSA as Birmingham is a densely populated city with a vast number of single-handed practitioners and no precedent for them to work together in ways that were beginning to be necessitated by the NHS reforms. However, it rapidly became apparent that housing an individual practice in the resource centre itself would be 'a bridge too far'. Such a move would effectively prevent surrounding practices from using the facility at all and so a decision was taken that the 'resident' staff would include a range of community nurses, paramedics and social services, but not GPs or their teams.

Local GPs needed to express sufficient initial interest to move forward with proposals and were asked to demonstrate a clear commitment before any building work began. It was proposed that the extent of their commitment to use the facility should be itemized by a contract document to be drawn up by the FHSA.

It was felt that there would be a greater chance of success if the pilot site was selected in an area from which access to major acute hospitals was relatively difficult, expensive or time-consuming. Reliance on public transport therefore became a major consideration.

In addition, it was determined that priority would be given to a site where an existing building could be adapted or extended at minimum cost and that there should be local community interest and support for the proposal.

Nevertheless the single most important criterion in selecting a site and in determining what should go into the centre was the wish to see services provided from this base which would begin to meet identified health needs within the population served. This meant that any site would need to have the scope for a flexible mix of different health and social care elements. An analysis by specialty was undertaken of the appropriateness and cost-efficiency of moving various types of outpatient clinics into a primary care resource centre. Ideally this should have included a structured survey of GPs and the systematic collation of hospital clinicians' views. In reality, it relied more closely on reports of similar types of service provision from elsewhere in the country.

The 'Building a Healthy Birmingham' team, as part of its planned relocation of hospital services, had already commissioned and completed work to identify the communities in the city with the longest public transport travelling times to existing acute units and those with the lowest rates of car ownership. The Community Unit had also previously undertaken detailed consultations with residents close to buildings which were already owned but which they would like to redevelop. Both these major pieces of work were accessible without any further investment and, as a result, it became clear reasonably quickly that there were two equally attractive possible locations. The only way to choose between these two was to test the all-important climate of GP opinion in the surrounding practices.

Testing GP opinion

All the GPs in each of the two localities were invited to meet to discuss the concept and the details of a primary care resource centre or to send along a representative of the practice such as the practice manager. The meetings were surprisingly well attended and it was rewarding to discover that there was

considerable interest in both locations. But one group seemed
more enthusiastic, less risk-aversive and slightly less daunted by
the prospect of collaboration with the FHSA. Hence Quinton
was selected.

Quinton is an area of Edgbaston with a largely indigenous
population and a high number of elderly people. It has pockets
of very considerable social and economic deprivation which
managers and planners can be blind to because of the relative
affluence of the rest of the area. In spite of this, the problems
are well recognized by those who live and work there, not least
because the existing clinic building was an exceedingly old and
dilapidated, prefabricated hut offering little that could be
described as 'enhanced'.

Information from the locality showed that Quinton had a
particularly high rate of inpatient admission for diabetes. This
was likely to reflect the high proportion of elderly people in the
population, but also raised questions about the scope for
improving the management of diabetes in the community.
Strengthening local diabetic care began to emerge as one of the
foremost objectives of the primary care resource centre for
Quinton. It would offer support for GPs wishing to provide a
higher standard of care for their own patients, consultant
expertise through 'master-classes' and specialized services such
as fundoscopy.

Outreach services

Over the months of planning a debate was taking place on
many levels about the outreaching of hospital services, probably because so many fundholders had chosen this model of
provision. Those who liked the idea or felt they were 'shaking
things up a little' talked of the advantages. Those who doubted
the cost-effectiveness or were, on principle, opposed to fundholding, talked only of a two-tier service or the erosion of the
critical hospital base. Ironically, fundholders in Birmingham –
who were unusually small in number – expressed a firm belief
that consultant clinics in their own practices were both undesirable and unnecessary. Undesirable because they uniformly
feared any further diminution in hospital provision and

unnecessary because Birmingham is compact and travel to hospital is reasonably easy from anywhere in the city.

Under pressure not simply to continue with planning for Quinton but to actually begin building, the concept of experimentation became the dominant theme. Quinton was going to provide an opportunity to test the value of outpatient clinics in local centres. The experiment would encompass a range of specialties and particular procedures, the choice of which would depend on an assessment of local need and a match between the interests of hospital clinicians and local GPs. It was necessary for GPs to accept some loss of choice of consultant and to generate enough patients to make local sessions worthwhile. The physical limitations of the proposed new building at Quinton also meant that only services which did not require large amounts of specialist equipment were going to be practical. A study of the literature and the known health needs of the city and the locality suggested the initial inclusion of orthopaedics, ophthalmology, antenatal care, mental illness and services for elderly people.

Less experimentally, physiotherapy, speech therapy, occupational therapy and chiropody were seen as high priorities for improvement at local level. Access to these services was seen by both GPs and community staff as a particular problem especially in relation to supporting elderly people living at home, following strokes or heart disease. The development of the primary health care resource centre was seen as an opportunity to provide these services more effectively from a facility shared by a number of GPs but without the threat of loss of patients which many GPs perceive as ever-present. These then seemed to be the most pressing needs in serving the population of Quinton. Beyond this it was hoped that a range of other services could be attracted into the resource centre including social services, other local authority services and voluntary organizations. A key test of the success of this model was expressed as the extent to which it provided a 'one-stop' access point for primary care. It was anticipated that its existence would improve communication and cross-agency working in the area. Box 3.1 is a list generated during the planning of the Quinton Centre of the features of a primary health care resource centre which would be considered to add value in some way.

Box 3.1: Value-adding features of a resource centre

- Decentralized diagnostic facilities
- Satellite outpatient clinics
- Facilitation of shared care e.g. diabetes, asthma
- Community physiotherapy, chiropody, nursing, health visiting
- Direct access to 'outreach' therapy sessions
- Location for mobile screening units
- Day theatre/treatment rooms for use by GPs or hospital 'outreach' staff
- Satellite dental surgery or resident dentist
- Training and teaching facilities
- Vision testing and audiometry
- Health promotion activities
- Bookable rooms for community groups
- Space to let for complementary medicine e.g. osteopathy

The centre is now open and is managed by South Birmingham Community Trust. Currently services include community health, midwifery, home care and social services. Specialist outreach services are being negotiated. Much work remains to be done to ensure that the Quinton Centre houses the most appropriate services, that the quality of service is enhanced and that other services or communities do not suffer disproportionately as a result of its development. Support has flagged least among the provider managers and this may be due to their pragmatic view that the very worst that could happen is that the good people of Quinton get a dramatically better health centre.

Others have argued that naming new facilities such as Quinton is merely window dressing and 'a rose by any other name would smell as sweet'. Certainly 'primary care resource centre' means very little to anyone, even those who work within the service. Nevertheless there is an argument for endeavouring to find a more meaningful and descriptive title. We should acknowledge that service users have a relatively clear concept of a hospital or a family doctor. It may be important that they understand the purpose of any new outlet or we may be resigning ourselves to years of future research into why these marvellous developments are underused or abused.

In fact, labelling has huge psychological importance. It is a well known phenomenon in medicine that patients often feel better if they are told the name of their illness. Perhaps those who worked on the Quinton Project, struggling to understand the purpose and the politics, trying to communicate across cultures and vastly different perspectives, and hoping to 'sell' an inadequately worked-up model of care to unconvinced and battle-weary professionals, would feel better if they had known that what they were doing was actually informal joint commissioning.

Service models for a primary care resource centre in Birmingham

Sarah Taylor

In the early stages of planning for what became the Quinton Primary Care Resource Centre, the project group considered a number of examples of the kinds of services that might be provided from a new 'local care facility'. Three of these are set out below. They were drafted as examples of the kind of 'concrete' service initiative which could turn Birmingham's primary care strategy into reality.

The strategy had been formulated to give balance to the largely hospital-based plans which had dominated NHS development in Birmingham over the previous decade. For many years primary care services had been left to their own devices with the resultant wide range of practice provision. There are examples of strong and visionary general medical practice. However, there is a continuing predominance of smaller practices and variable and fragmented relationships between general practice and community health services. Many GPs regard the FHSA in a threatening light. The main aims of the strategy were to take all stakeholders along in its development, to build on the positive aspects of primary care in Birmingham, and to work with motivated practitioners to bring about change. Local care facilities, or resource centres, were an important part of the plan.

The project group had begun by exploring opportunities for shifting traditional secondary care. It rapidly became clear, however, that if any service developments were to be significantly different to previous experiments they would have to develop the primary care model itself, and change practice as well as structure or location of services. Local care facilities were one option which was given added impetus by being seen as off-shoot investment of the major hospital changes being planned for the city.

A number of examples were developed of the services which might be provided from a new centre. The three described here are diabetic services, services for elderly people and ophthalmology. They give an indication of the number of patients needed to make the service viable in an area with 10–15 general practitioners and a population of 20–30 000 people. The criteria on which they were based include:

- a primary care focus – to be innovative and imaginative about the services which could be provided from the community setting

- a focus for multi-disciplinary team-working so that services would be chosen which benefited from being provided collaboratively

- to encourage a shift from the centralized secondary sector where services could be more appropriately and effectively provided locally

- to give a community focus to the area in which it was sited

- to give an opportunity to invest across a number of GP practices as well as in local community services
- to be shaped according to local need.

Diabetes service

The model proposes a primary care/GP-based service and is a move away from the hospital/consultant led approach towards the concept of district diabetic centres. The service would consist of:

- GPs running disease management and health promotion clinics
- support from nurse specialists based at the centre
- community nursing services
- chiropody, dietitians, health education
- direct access to on-site diagnostic and investigative pathology, including optometry.

Diabetes is known to affect 1.5–2% of the population (up to 5% in some sub-groups) of which up to half are undiagnosed. Therefore the proposed pilot serving 10–15 GPs with a population of 20–30 000 people would expect to find between 300–600 diabetics, one in four of whom is insulin dependent. Two or three new cases could expect to be referred per week.

There is good evidence of the effectiveness both of control of diabetes itself, foot and skin care, and prevention of complications, including eye disease. This model could therefore be worked up as a pilot for working with local clinicians on patterns of care, guidelines for local practice in the use of generalist and specialist services, health promotion and disease management. There is the potential for a changed pattern of diabetic service in the city.

Services for elderly people

The centre could act as a focus for:

- geriatricians

- out-patient clinics

- community-based chiropody and physiotherapy, currently under-resourced and inadequate

- liaison between community nurses, GPs, consultants, practice nurses

- stroke rehabilitation

- health promotion activities

- local authority and voluntary services.

The pilot elderly resource centres presently being run in Birmingham, e.g. in Selly Oak, could be used as a model. They bring together community-based resource teams from health, social services and the voluntary sector with pump-priming monies from joint finance. Their task is to identify the needs of elderly people and their carers within a neighbourhood. There is direct access to the teams and they also take referrals from primary care professionals. They access and provide services covering physical and mental health, self care, social relationships, communication, accommodation, financial and emotional support and advice.

Ophthalmology

Joint protocols for the management of eye diseases agreed by ophthalmologists and general practitioners would encourage appropriate referrals at the appropriate time, and screening and early detection to prevent eye disease, particularly glaucoma and diabetic retinopathy.

Two per cent of 60-year-olds and over 40% of those over 80 years of age suffer from senile cataract. In an area of 10–15 GPs with a population of 20–30 000 people, one would expect 700 people with cataracts sufficiently severe to disturb their eyesight, and between 70–90 people developing cataract for the first time each year. Glaucoma probably affects about 70 people in this GP area (0.5% of people aged between 55–60 and over 4% of those over 80 years). About a quarter of these have other affected family members and can therefore be identified as high risk and entitled to free eye testing. The loss of vision caused by glaucoma can be reduced by early detection and treatment. GPs, optometrists and ophthalmologists working together can achieve this.

Examples such as these formed the starting point for a whole series of meetings with general practitioners and hospital clinicians to consider the kinds of services that might be provided from a new centre. It was at this point that the politics of the health service in Birmingham and the West Midlands intervened. The Regional Health Authority (RHA) raised the profile of the project by identifying capital to be spent on high profile primary care developments and the regional chairman intervened, looking for something concrete on which to wield a bulldozer. This speeded up the timetable and brought about a rather pragmatic decision on which site to choose, based on the enthusiasm of the GPs consulted, and the capital feasibility of adapting current community services' facilities.

The decision on services, based on the discussions with doctors, was to concentrate on care of the elderly, ophthalmology and optometrist services, diabetic services, dermatology, ear, nose and throat services (especially for children), rheumatology and soft tissue disorders.

The centre is now a reality. An operational policy is in place which brings together a range of health and social care staff. But this is only a beginning. Contracts and joint protocols have to be negotiated and much remains to be done to commission and manage the new kinds of services envisaged by the project group.

A resource centre without walls

Maggie Jee

One of the early decisions of the Croydon Community Health Trust was to organize a new nursing neighbourhood to be coterminous with the effective catchment area of three GP practices clustered together in the north of the borough. The ambition was to radically enhance the possibilities for collaboration of the GP practices and community services. To this end, a neighbourhood office-base was set up adjacent to the practices, and a neighbourhood manager appointed, with a delegated budget and a brief to support co-ordinated activities. At the same time, a monthly lunchtime meeting was instituted to which all staff in the practices and neighbourhood were invited. The London Road Health Co-operative (LRHC) was born.

A new set of relationships was fostered, that would allow staff in the different agencies to work together much more closely than before. As a result of this imaginative restructuring, many services, resources and protocols are now shared, and all staff are known to each other and have regular opportunities to meet together to assess joint practice and plan new initiatives. Although no one involved in its setting up would have thought of it in this way, the LRHC has become a kind of 'resource centre without walls'.

Origins

The initial idea for the LRHC was developed by a keen GP and the chief executive of the Croydon Community Health Trust. It arose at a time of rapid change in the health service. Transformations in primary care meant that the various health professionals in the area were facing a great variety of challenges, but were also being presented with a number of new opportunities for collaboration.

The three GP practices concerned were well established in the locality, but knew each other only slightly – they had shared an off-duty rota for 50 years and had traditionally gathered for Christmas drinks, but there was little further contact. All were wondering what the future held for them. They were having to adjust to the new contract and facing the need to make the most economical use of resources. Fundholding was on the horizon.

Geography, too, made it sense for them to get together. Their proximity – two of the practices are literally opposite each other, the third is only 100 yards up the road – make these practices the obvious 'health centre', of their area. The population they serve is largely working-class, fairly stable, and with a higher than average proportion of young families. It has many of the problems of the inner city, including unemployment, homelessness, and drug addiction.

The practices had all enjoyed good relationships with community services. In 1990, the Croydon Community Health Trust was established. With its strong and enthusiastic leadership, and energetic team, the trust had what could be characterized as a 'hands off' or 'freeing-up' management style. Its corporate philosophy embraced a concern to find opportunities to improve professional relationships with GPs, and hence patient services. The trust was very keen to organize a nursing neighbourhood around a cluster of practices as a structure in which participants could innovate. Box 3.2 shows the staff involved.

Box 3.2: London Road Health Co-operative: personnel

3 GP practices		1 CHS neighbourhood	
GPs	11	neighbourhood manager	1
(1 × 3, 1 × 3, 1 × 5)		clerks	2
receptionists	18	school nurses	2
practice managers	3	district nursing teams	12
practice nurses	9	(4 × DNs, 4 × ENs,	
		3 × NAs, 1 × CSN)	
counsellors	4	physiotherapists	1
		optometrist	1
		chiropodist	1
		community midwives	3
Total	**45**	**Total**	**23**

Setting up the LRHC

The trust
Prior to the formation of the LRHC, the community services staff attached to the three GP practices were split between

different neighbourhoods with different managers. The organization of the new neighbourhood, and the setting up of the office-base, involved all staff in quite an upheaval. Never-the-less, it was done with great enthusiasm and high expectations.

The GP practices

The GP practices, too, were enthusiastic about this reorganization since they could see the potential benefits of having their nursing teams linked under the same nurse manager, with the further advantage of having their office-base on-site. Unlike the trust though, the GPs were involved in no major reorganization of staff or premises (though one practice had to find space for their health visitors). What was required of the GPs was more a reorganization of their ideas and attitudes: they had to learn to think and work collaboratively.

Philosophy and practice

The three practices willingly supported an informal agreement to work closely with each other (with the proviso that they would retain their own identities and practice philosophies). However, it was not spelt out in detail what becoming a 'cooperative' would mean. Nevertheless, the overall aim seemed fairly straightforward: all health professionals, irrespective of their management structure, would try to work more closely together to improve services for their patients. Absolutely nothing was imposed. No 'outsider' – FHSA, Trust, or Act of Parliament – had said, or could say, 'You will do this!' Moreover, although two 'key workers' (the neighbourhood manager and one of the senior GPs) were going to take a lead, no special facilitator or project leader was appointed. It was up to the group to find its own way.

What has been achieved?

- Community services initiatives have drawn in GPs. As a result, GPs are learning to use community services' resources more appropriately.

- GPs are increasingly cooperating across practices, and are thereby becoming a potential resource for each other.

- Team-building initiatives are providing a psychological resource. In a supportive environment, all co-op members become a resource for each other.

Over a period of two and a half years a variety of small-scale projects have been set up that have enabled the practices and the neighbourhood to work more closely together. In fact, few of these projects are wholly new, and most are primarily nursing or community services' initiatives. They are a long way short of integrated clinical practice, and they clearly illustrate the resilience of the barriers to be overcome.

Nevertheless, they represent significant improvements. On the whole, trust staff are doing what they have always done, but now they are bringing the GPs along too. As a result, GPs have acquired a much better understanding of the roles and functions of trust staff, and the services they provide. What makes the LRHC initiative particularly encouraging is the growing involvement of GPs with neighbourhood activities, the importance given to democratic team-building initiatives, and the adoption of policies and practices that are consistent across the neighbourhood.

GPs have also learnt about, and from, each other, and this has further enabled them to agree to support some consistent approaches to patient care across the neighbourhood, and even to initiate their own cross-practice proposals.

For the sake of exposition, these achievements are distinguished here as either operational or team-building in nature. In practice they are enmeshed. Several initiatives could not have taken place without good communications and a high degree of team integration, and team identity has been forged through the implementation of some of the activities.

Operational achievements

- An integrated community nursing team (one which includes district nurses and their teams, health visitors, school nurses and midwives) works consistently across the three GP practices.

- Physiotherapy, chiropody and optometry services are provided on-site for the patients of all three practices. Each practice hosts one therapy.

GPs have become much more knowledgeable about these therapies. They have learnt what different services offer, how to use them efficiently, and how to negotiate changes to get the service they want. GPs have also learnt how to share these resources. Initially, they were somewhat anxious about what might happen if their patients visited the other practices; but they have coped, and no patients have been tempted to change practices.

- A standardized palliative care box, agreed by the whole co-op, is used by all district nurse teams in the homes of terminally ill patients.

- All district nurses are provided with stock-prescription items to prevent delays and cut down on unnecessary demands on GPs.

- All nurses and doctors follow the same protocol for the diagnosis and treatment of leg ulcers. This protocol is regularly audited by the co-op.

The leg ulcer protocol started as a community services' nursing initiative but has since been taken up by GPs too. One GP has completed the recognized training course and now participates in cascade training sessions. Most of the co-op's GPs and nurses have attended these sessions.

- Health visitors run a 'drop-in' mother-and-toddler group for vulnerable parents from all three practices.

The three practices are very involved in this community services'/health visitors' initiative, which they part fund. As a result, they have come to understand and value the health educational and support functions of health visitors.

- The three practices are negotiating to open a new shared site which will house complementary therapies and provide a venue for cross-practice patient groups, counselling, and voluntary sector groups.

GPs say they have found on-site therapies provided by community services, and the health visitors' 'drop-in' (together with counselling, which is currently offered by two practices), so beneficial to patients and patient care that they see great scope for extending these services.

- The three practices are developing joint health promotion initiatives in line with *Health of the Nation* targets, which involve all staff.

- A quarterly patients' newsletter, *Health Matters,* containing advice and health information, is written and produced by representatives from each practice and the neighbourhood, and it has won a health education award.

Team-building achievements
A monthly lunchtime co-op meeting, open to all, generates, discusses and plans new initiatives, tackles problems and provides a social venue. This meeting has always been integral to the idea of how the co-op would function. The other meetings, groups and activities, outlined below, have developed from this monthly forum as the co-op has felt the need for more structure. The co-op meeting also acts as a valuable psychological resource, pulling people together in a supportive environment.

- Monthly meetings of the planning group develop detailed plans for discussion and agreement by the whole co-op.

- Smaller working groups develop specific ideas and projects (e.g. the *Health Matters* newsletter, health promotion).

- A co-op constitution has been agreed to aid decision-making and implementation of projects, and to clarify roles.

- A co-op year-plan is being developed with specific targets and time limits.

- Two study days have been held for all co-op members, with virtually all staff attending (58 out of 60 staff attended the second study day). These have significantly enhanced team-building.

- Cascade training sessions are organized to spread good practice efficiently and effectively.

Difficulties

None of these achievements have been easy. It must be remembered that the LRHC example is set in an environment of good will, where a strong, innovative community services trust is prepared to meet GPs more than half way, and where a group of GPs are willing to make an effort too. Even so, progress can be painfully slow. Although the points that follow are particular to the LRHC, they also have a more general application. Many will arise in any setting or structure where health professionals with very different practices, philosophies, contractual obligations and financial interests are encouraged to share resources.

Initial differences among the three practices and the neighbourhood

At the start of the co-op, the GP practices and the trust were at very different stages of development, and embraced quite different approaches and philosophies. In addition, the parties did not know each other as well as they had assumed. As a result, they did not realize they were all at different levels – a fact which only emerged slowly as they tried to work together. This undoubtedly caused some friction.

In terms of integrated working, for instance, the trust was ahead of all three practices. District nurses, health visitors and managers are all used to working collaboratively in teams, and to taking initiatives in seeking new ways of delivering services. Indeed, the GPs were all relatively new to the idea of teamwork, were developing their understanding of the primary health care team, and not all of them had regular practice meetings. They were certainly not used to meeting together across the practices and there were no precedents for working together.

Slow pace of change and development

From some points of view, the LRHC can seem a lumbering great thing. The LRHC has no facilitator, and struggles to work as a democratic, non-hierarchical group. Frustration may be caused when some considerable time is spent with discussions going round in circles.

Tensions between GPs and neighbourhood

Some neighbourhood staff have felt that the trust's and the neighbourhood's contribution have been greater than the uneven commitment of GPs. They experienced a major upheaval, yet the pace of progress towards more collaborative approaches to patient care seems very slow.

During the life of the co-op it has become clear that even the most willing GPs do not fully understand how community services work, the range of services they provide, or the individual roles of staff. In the early days of the co-op this led to confusion and misunderstanding.

Joint protocols are not easy to enforce in a non-contractual environment. Whereas community services staff can be given clear instructions about leg ulcer treatments, GPs are entitled to continue to pursue their own procedures, and their practice nurses must comply.

Tension among GPs

As independent contractors, GPs are not used to consulting each other or working together. There are few precedents for GPs to follow (except where there is an obvious benefit, such as being united in a struggle against poor hospital services).

At various times during the development of the co-op it was unclear where the boundaries of responsibility to the co-op lay. As a result, individual practices sometimes treated as purely private matters, events, changes or decisions that were to have a powerful effect on the whole co-op, which would better have been discussed with all parties.

What can we learn from LRHC?

The LRHC is essentially a voluntary collaboration between community health services and a small cluster of GP practices. Any similar attempts to set up a 'resource centre without walls' are likely to encounter many of the same issues.

- Even when GPs are eager to see changes, community services will have to make most of the running.

- In the absence of contractual obligations, a collaborative venture of the LRHC sort can only be as strong and successful as the interpersonal relationships that exist between the parties – a hazardously ephemeral business.

- If such an informally-constituted, mixed group is given voluntary, democratic process, without strong leadership or a facilitator, progress may be made at a snail's pace.

- Managers cannot just take a good idea (such as resource-sharing) to GPs and expect it to be taken up and work smoothly. GPs generally have little or no experience of sharing things except within their own practices (and even this can be problematic), let alone across practices. They may have misunderstandings about the roles of community staff and the services they provide, so would not be clear about what they were being offered and/or expected to share. Many GPs do not work as well with community services as those at London Road clearly did.

- It is thus extremely difficult to harness the energy, ideas and good will of keen, independent contractors. Ultimately GPs will only do what they want to do. But committed, clever and patient community services staff can bring about change by gradually and subtly influencing GPs' attitudes. It is very hard work, even with willing GPs.

- However, the task is made very much easier if community services have something that GPs want – they will then be prepared to come on board relatively quickly and this may help to convince GPs elsewhere in the locality to cooperate, overcoming doubts, even about such apparently radical practices as referring patients to surgeries other than their own. Those GPs who see how community services can indeed enhance their own work will certainly want to make the most effective use of community staff.

Polyclinics – an alternative to practice-based care? 4

Franklin Apfel and Pearl Brown

Introduction

The British model of general practice, with its emphasis on personal responsibility for patients, comprehensiveness and continuity of care, has not been surpassed in any other health care system. But not everyone gets a good service from family-based practice which relies on a fairly stable population registered with a general practitioner. The diverse and mobile populations of our cities, in particular, pose challenges for those providing primary care services.

Cities have immensely varied cultural and racial neighbourhoods. Their residents may be securely housed or temporary visitors. They may be students or refugees or homeless families or people who travel into the city each day to work. As parts of cities decay there are more people who have few choices and feel trapped by poverty, poor housing, poor employment prospects and social isolation. To respond appropriately to the differing community needs of city neighbourhoods, primary care itself has to be diverse. It needs to adapt and extend and to become more flexible to ensure high quality services for those who do not want or do not fit into family-based practice. Polyclinics, with a range of walk-in services and specialist clinics, have been proposed as an alternative. In this chapter Franklin Apfel discusses the characteristics of polyclinics and urgent care centres with examples from Europe and the USA and Pearl Brown describes the development of a new service in South Westminster, London.

Like the resource centres in the previous chapter, the Westminster Centre is a capital-led development. It is a planned response to the closure of a local hospital and the acknowledged weakness of primary care in the neighbourhood. Its aims are to compensate for these deficiencies by extending the range of care available outside hospital buildings. Like the resource centres, there are numerous ways of interpreting these aims and of judging success. Again, the importance and complexity of 'working the boundaries' are very clear. Negotiating between generalists and specialists and between numerous agencies becomes the main management task.

Polyclinics and urgent care centres

Franklin Apfel

An organizational framework

In principle, polyclinics offer great potential for integrating health services in a primary care setting. Polyclinics bring together several providers under one physical or conceptual roof. These providers may bridge the ground between specialists and generalists and bring in community care social services.

The polyclinic as an organizational framework can be usefully classified by the extent to which providers share services and function within a managed environment (Box 4.1).

In its simplest form, Type A, a polyclinic is a shared office complex, a building where several practitioners provide services, in parallel, under one roof. Such clustering of providers is convenient for patients and allows for informal networking of providers. However, such office complexes frequently duplicate services like reception, waiting, and record keeping, and offer purchasers few efficiencies.

Box 4.1: Polyclinic typology

A Shared office complex

- common building
- shared maintenance

B Shared services

- reception
- record storage
- diagnostic services
- education
- transport
- creche

C Managed systems

- strategic planning
- resource allocation
- determining priorities
- contract negotiations
- peer review audit

D Without walls

- agreed management systems
- separate services

Efficiencies can be realized when providers in polyclinics begin to share services such as a central reception, waiting, laboratory, X-ray, and other ancillary service as in Type B. Such centralized provision of support, treatment such as minor surgery, and diagnostic services enhance the scope of the centre and the capacities of providers. However, start-up costs for such centres are significant.

Shared premises and services do not necessarily influence the professional's method of practice. Managed polyclinic systems, Type C can influence professional behaviours. In such centres behaviours are modified by engaging professionals in:

- strategic decision-making e.g. resource allocation, developmental prioritizing

- peer review and audit

- improved clinical communications e.g. shared patient records, protocols, internal referrals

- active participation in contracting e.g. organized input to purchasers.

Such managed systems should lead to improved quality of care as well as yielding economic efficiencies.

Type D are polyclinics without walls. These polyclinics consist of separate services bound together through agreed management arrangements. While physically separate, these 'hamlets' may realize many of the benefits of managed centres without the need for high initial capital expenditures.

Advantages and disadvantages

Polyclinics offer patients convenient access to a number of services and a choice of physician (Box 4.2). Sharing premises, facilities and back-up services offer providers lower costs, and also staff get more scope for peer review. Gains for purchasers include increased provider competition, lower operating costs, and more flexibility in the use of resources.

Box 4.2: Polyclinics – advantages and disadvantages

	Advantages	**Disadvantages**
Patient	greater access greater choice greater convenience less waiting time	depersonalization fragmentation excess referrals
Provider	greater clinical time greater peer review greater expanded scope less cost from shared premises and administration	loss of independence deskilling
Purchaser	greater resource flexibility greater competition greater choice less operating costs	start-up costs duplication

---

On the downside, patients may feel the service is fragmented and depersonalized. It is also possible they receive more treatment than necessary. Doctors may feel less independent and may become deskilled because of the ease of referral. Effective administration of polyclinics requires designated skilled managers. Purchasers' problems include high start up costs especially for free-standing centres.

The polyclinic system in the Czech Republic

The Czech Republic spends roughly the same proportion of its gross national product on health services as the UK (Table 4.1). While currently undergoing rapid and extensive reform, the Czech health system, until recently, was based on a Soviet style hierarchy of polyclinics.

The basic service unit was a community or workplace mini-polyclinic. Providers included nurses, general practitioners (list size 1500–2500), paediatricians (list size 1100), gynaecologists (list size 600), and stomatologists (list size 2500). Practitioners provided domiciliary and out-of-hours service. After-hours calls in urban areas went to a central station and a GP or paediatrician was dispatched to patients' homes or patients

Table 4.1: Czech–UK health care comparisons

	CSFR	UK
% GNP	5.8	6.0
Hospital days per capita	2.3	2.1
Outpatients visits per capita	14.7	4.5
Beds per 100 000 population	126	68
Life expectancy	F = 75.3	F = 78.4
	M = 67.7	M = 72.7
Infant mortality	11.9	9
Physicians per 100 000 population	37	17
	(F = 55%)	

Source: *Who-Euro Database* (1990–1)

transported to accident and emergency units. In rural areas physicians provided after-hour services on a scheduled rota basis.

The average number of outpatient visits per year was a striking 14.7 per capita (UK, 4.5). First level provider referral rates to hospital-based and secondary level specialists ranged up to 85%. This high rate of referral is explained in part by:

• public and professional perception of hospital care as best

• public demand, backed up at times with gifts for speedy referral

• inadequate resourcing of providers e.g. lack of continuing training, minimal diagnostic equipment

• progressive de-skilling of providers due to low status of community-based providers and the ease and expectation of referral

• under-resourcing of specialty providers in non-hospital based polyclinics, requiring referral to hospital-based providers for surgical care.

On the positive side, care or at least initial evaluation, was accessible and free of charge to all citizens close to home. There were 37 physicians per 100 000 population (UK, 17). Minimal waiting lists existed for specialty evaluation and treatment.

On the downside, in spite of widely available polyclinics, the system was still very focused on hospital care. The Czech health system has 126 beds per 100 000 population (UK, 68). Patients had limited choice of physician and often experienced depersonalized care. Privileges were granted to certain social and political groups with discrimination against others. Centralized planning did not necessarily reflect local needs and preferences, nor did it allow for the development of local management capacities.

Urgent care centres in California

In the 1980s, in Sacramento County, the Emergency Center (sic) was open from 8 am to midnight, every day. It offered

X-rays and many lab tests, and treated abdominal pain, eye injuries, burns, fractures, pneumonia, 'flu, neck and back injuries, as well as sore throats, ear infections, lacerations, sprains and bruises. No appointment was needed, patients were seen within 30–60 minutes (Box 4.3).

When people needing urgent attention do not have a good GP service, urgent care centres may offer a 'stopgap' solution. They may be open at all times. They may be situated more locally than a hospital. Commuters, tourists and others without a regular GP can use them.

Convenience can be a major factor for patients. They may also get better access to emergency care and more scope for diagnosis and treatment than many GPs offer. The schemes

---

Box 4.3: The Emergency Center

Hours	The Emergency Center is open from 8 am to midnight, every day, including weekends and holidays.
Services available	X-rays and many lab. tests can be carried out at the Center. Almost any acute injury or illness can be treated, including:

lacerations	fractures
'flu	pneumonia
sprains	bruises
abdominal pain	neck and back injuries
eye injuries	sore throats
burns	ear infections

The Center also undertakes pre-employment and driver's physical exams.

Life-threatening injury or illness is best treated in the nearest hospital emergency room.

Using the Emergency Center	No appointment is needed. The injured or ill person may be brought without prior notification. Following examination and treatment, the Center will determine the person's ability to return to work.

Box 4.4: Urgent care centres – advantages and disadvantages

	Advantages	**Disadvantages**
Patient	• greater access • greater scope • greater convenience	• episodic care • not connected to other services • medical model
Provider	• low entry capital • better life style • income maintained	• longer hours • non-mainstream • isolation
Purchaser	• plug gaps • reduced costs compared to A & E • choice	• greater start-up costs • threat to A & E survival

enable purchasers to plug gaps in the system of cover for emergencies more cheaply than by providing full accident and emergency services. In California schemes such as this have stimulated some GPs to themselves provide the services that meet the needs that such centres were fulfilling.

Urgent care centres offer little scope for consideration of psychological or social dimensions to patients' problems – the medical model prevails. Although some patients may welcome the simple 'in/out' treatment, such episodic care may not be ideal from a public health point of view. Practitioners can become quite isolated from the mainstream health care system. Purchasers may find start-up costs considerable.

Experiments with urgent care centres, minor trauma units or minor injuries centres are now taking place in many UK cities and offer an alternative to hospital accident and emergency departments. But if local general practice is good, improving it still further, with extra training and equipment, may be a better use of resources.

South Westminster Centre for Health, London

Pearl Brown

The certain closure of Westminster Hospital and the poor primary care services in South Westminster promoted great local concern. The response by Riverside Community Healthcare NHS Trust was to create a centre which would integrate health and social care and bring together community services with some acute services; £1.7 million was spent converting a three-story former nurses' home.

The centre contains two GP practices, a pharmacy, walk-in nurse practitioner services, phlebotomy, facilities for minor surgery and space for voluntary organizations and advice agencies – all on the ground floor. On the first floor are X-ray and ultrasound, 15 consultant outpatient clinics, plus venous ulcer clinics, physiotherapy, speech therapy, occupational therapy, dental care, chiropody and dietetics. The new local academic department of general practice has some space there along with osteopathy, acupuncture and therapeutic massage. A toy library, Age Concern, Crawlers' Clubs, an Alzheimer's support group and Befriend a Family also use the first floor. At the top of the building are health visitors and district nursing staff, administration staff and a local authority (Westminster) social services team for children and families.

The project has taken time to reach its full potential. Six months after opening, much remained to be worked out, such as protocols for X-ray, whether GPs would be able to refer patients at once to specialists if they happened to be in the building, and so on. But the conversion was well done and patients liked the building. Lessons learned in managing the creation of the centre included:

• planning takes time – important to cling on to the vision

• revisit original philosophy – often

• involve GPs early – ask them what they want in the centre and do not rely on the FHSA to find GPs

- engage purchasers' interest

- involve local community – joint finance-funded worker helped for two years

- develop a public relations strategy – good notices and local publicity

- identify ownership and accountability for all services – especially with consultants

- funding responsibilities – these involve much negotiation e.g. should the FHSA be funding the nurse practitioners?

- get a clear brief on what information purchasers want – likely to show concern about high start-up costs and capitation difficulties in transition period, before acute services shed costs

- keep the local authority on your side.

To sum up, strong management is needed to keep everyone involved and feeling committed. People have to share the vision and much work is needed to get people working together in new ways.

There have been minor difficulties in making the centre accessible for health professionals and in the smooth introduction of all the facilities and clinics. Some clinics were not well supported and lines of decision-making were not as clear as they should have been, but many of the problems were being resolved after the first few months. The centre is showing promising progress. The nurse practitioners' minor treatment centre (MTC), for example, is proving increasingly popular with local people (Box 4.5).

Nurse practitioner service

Local distress about the loss of the local accident & emergency service, plus concern about some poor quality general practice in the vicinity, promoted the setting up of the nurse practitioner service.

Within the first nine months attendances rose from an average of 179 to 324 per month. The minor treatment centre was

---

Box 4.5: Nurse practitioner service – minor treatment centre

- Health information and advice
- Health promotion
- Women's health, family planning
- Support and counselling
- Pre- and post-operative advice
- Minor injuries and accidents
- Access and referral to other local services
- Dressings and injections
- Limited list of drugs

---

originally open from Monday to Friday, 9.00 am to 6.00 pm, and soon extended to Saturday mornings and then to Sundays as well. Weekday times extended, from 8 am to 8 pm. It offers a walk-in service staffed by experienced nurses who see anyone who lives or works locally, and can advise, assess, treat or refer (Table 4.2).

Table 4.2: Attendances at nurse practitioner service

Month	Average/day	Average/week	Average/month
May	16.04	58.00	290
June	20.00	75.20	296
July	28.25	106.25	425
August	26.00	99.25	397
Local residents		77%	
Reg. local GPs		80%	
Reg. outside		11%	
Not registered		8%	
Under 16		15%	
16–64		60%	
65 +		25%	

Initial studies on attendances after one year found:

- 234 clients said they would have attended their GP if the MTC had not been available. Of these, 60 were referred to a GP and 166 were managed by a nurse practitioner

- the pressure is also being taken off casualty services by the MTC. Ninety five clients said they would have attended a casualty department if one had been close by. After assessment, only ten of the 95 were referred to casualty

- an increasing number of clients, 27%, are returning to use the service with a new health problem

- Forty two per cent of clients are referred by GP surgeries, 19% come by word of mouth, and 16% work locally

- the convenient walk-in, no appointment facility was an important reason for attendance by 65% of clients and the nurse practitioners' service was first choice for 28%. Only 2% came because they could not get a GP appointment and 1% because they were not registered with a local GP.

Centre opening times

Planning permission for opening hours was limited originally due to anxiety by the local residents that the centre might prove to be a nuisance to them. Now the trust has won their support in gaining permission for opening 14 hours a day, seven days a week. This change in favour of the centre indicates that it is now viewed as a valuable asset by the local community.

GP practices

Two GP practices have operated five-days-a-week branch surgeries from the centre since November 1993. There is a separate entrance and both have attractive, well-appointed waiting areas for patients.

The GPs have made good use of the many services available at the centre. Forty two per cent of all attendances come from

GPs. The practice managers are part of the team which is looking at the integration of services and day-to-day organizational issues. One GP works regularly with the nurse practitioners to review the MTC walk-in clinic's attendance and services. Seven other local GPs from four practices, who provide a deputizing service for each other, hold their Saturday surgery at the centre.

Community groups

The centre is also proving very popular with community groups and the local residents association now holds its monthly meetings there.

Local voluntary groups which have established services include the Pimlico Toy Library and Befriend a Family. Also community development work has led to the formation of a number of self-help groups including the South Westminster and Pimlico Carers Support Group and the Mums Information and Support Group.

X-ray

GPs operating from the centre and other practices in the area have shown a great interest in the X-ray facility. In its first 12 weeks of operation, attendances more than doubled. It has proved a valuable addition to the centre's facilities as local people do not have to travel considerable distances to units in the major hospitals. Agreement has also been reached on the nurse practitioners being able to refer direct to X-ray.

Outpatients

The centre is now responding well to local demand for outpatient clinics. Consultants from the Chelsea and Westminster Hospital now run 16 separate outpatient clinics at the South Westminster Centre. These include ante-natal, dermatology,

ENT, seven medical clinics, two surgical clinics, two paediatric clinics and a gynaecology clinic. GPs can now send referral letters direct to the South Westminster Centre which is linked to the Patient Administrative Systems (PAS) at the hospital. This allows receptionists to make appointments for clinics on either site.

After consultation with local GPs, it was decided to include orthopaedics and gynaecology and to extend the diabetic service. Although GP involvement in the range of clinics to be provided was initiated a little late, such action can be reversed rapidly.

Planning groups

At the planning stage of the centre, several multidisciplinary groups were invited to plan services around care groups. With the delay of the building for one year and with staff changes, most of these groups lapsed. They are now being resurrected to ensure that the centre is not just a building with a number of disparate services. An example is the children's group whose main goal is to provide a focus for promoting good multi-disciplinary working, as well as to ensure that it can be accessed by GPs in the area. Its task is also to consider future development of services for children within the centre. Its members are mainly providers of children's services within the centre including child-psychology, child and adolescent mental health, the children and family social services team, community health visiting services, a community consultant paediatrician and a speech therapist. The first priority has been to develop operational policies for each service. Each representative produced a description of their services and the method by which they take referrals. This proved a useful starting tool for exchanging information and developing protocols.

Access

Access to the centre was not given as much priority and planned as well in advance as it might have been and working with the local authority to find solutions has been slow. It is vital to work with the local authority early on in the project planning stage. Although the physical access into the centre meets all the latest standards, other important access issues have emerged. These are:

- *Signage.* Finding the South Westminster Centre for Health has not always been easy. Westminster City Council turned down initial requests for street signs but has now relented and there will be local pedestrian signage.

- *Parking for GPs and consultants.* After considerable discussion with the local authority, one GP parking place has been agreed. Normally parking for GPs is only permitted at the principal practice location. At present, there are no reserved parking spaces for consultants, however, negotiations are continuing with Westminster City Council and local organizations.

- *Buses.* The Hoppa bus service, which links the centre with Chelsea and Westminster Hospital and Pimlico, stops nearby. But many potential users were not aware of its operation because there was not a designated bus stop. Bus stops, with timetables, will now be provided in local streets.

- *Patient transport service ambulance.* A minibus collects patients from their homes in Pimlico to attend the leg ulcer and chiropody clinics at the centre. Ambulances booked via Chelsea and Westminster Hospital are now provided for local people attending clinics. In the centre's first year the hospital's ambulance contract was not amended to include the centre and this omission was of great concern to the local public and GPs alike.

Conclusion

The centre continues to grow. The future looks promising. Shared care clinics between GPs and consultants are planned; paediatric physiotherapy and expanded adult services are to be introduced. A needle exchange and community psychiatric nursing service are to be developed by the local mental health trust. A hospice in the neighbouring district is planning to develop pain control clinics at the centre and the minor surgery unit, which initially had limited appeal to local general practice, is now growing in popularity.

The lessons that have been learned about opening and running a centre such as this are that a strong management structure is needed to continually review activities, to build on knowledge all the time, and not be afraid of changing and remodelling services as the need arises. The centre is owned and managed by the community trust. Three different trusts now work in the building and the collaboration between them has led to beneficial spin-offs in other parts of the district.

Hospital care at home   5

Liz Haggard and Egbert Bosma

Introduction

In this chapter we consider two of the ways in which traditional hospital services can be shifted into high quality care in the home. Liz Haggard discusses 'hospital-at-home' and Egbert Bosma describes an institute for pioneering new forms of home-based care in the Netherlands.

Hospital care at home is the term used to describe schemes which bring into the home intensive levels of care associated with acute hospitals, supplying medical, nursing and rehabilitation services as well as social support and equipment. In her review of developments in home care Marks describes it as 'the deliberate and planned relocation of hospital-style services and equipment into a home setting.[1] This may be an alternative to hospital admission or a means of reducing length of stay in hospital by providing continuing care after discharge. It is not simply an extension of the trend towards earlier discharge from hospital, or a way of reducing demand on hospital beds, or a short-term, cost-cutting exercise. Some schemes provide extremely specialized high technology care. All hospital care at home programmes represent a new way of thinking about the balance between home and hospital care.[2] They can be seen as an extension of primary care or as an extension of secondary care. As part of the current drive to shift services out of hospitals, the so-called substitution agenda, primary care strategy documents now frequently contain plans for hospitals-at-home. These come after a long, slow start in this country where the first scheme began in Peterborough almost 20 years ago.

Broadly, there are two organizational models for hospitals at home. One is the creation of a specialized team, usually hospital-based, often linked to a surgical specialty, which may seek to involve primary and community health staff. Examples are the Community Orthopaedic Project in Essex (COPE) and the support team for patients with HIV, based at St Mary's Hospital in London.[3,4] The other model which is described here by Liz Haggard, is a community-based service for a defined geographical population. It can be argued that in cities it is this model which could have the potentially greater impact on the balance of services. In major cities, in particular, with all the complexities of acute hospital providers, community-based, hospital-at-home schemes organized geographically and taking referrals from multiple acute providers, could offer an attractive alternative to hospital care.

Hospital-at-home schemes make people anxious. GPs are reluctant to take responsibility for someone discharged straight from an intensive care unit. Surgeons fear unanticipated complications and the impossibility of getting a patient back to the hospital in time. Managers realize it will not work without tight and quick liaison between hospital and community staff, doctors and nurses. Patients and their families want accurate backup information and a 24-hour telephone service. And yet in some parts of the country it works well and everyone seems satisfied.

One of the main lessons from the South Derbyshire case study is the need for rigorous definition of what is meant by hospital-at-home. Liz Haggard and her colleagues took every opportunity to repeat and to emphasize that theirs was a new ward, based in the community, and like every other ward had limited places, discharge procedures as formal as any other, targets for length of stay, was served by specialists as well as generalists, and required sufficient resources.[5] As for anxieties, they soon learned that staff were more likely to believe colleagues than managers. As part of the start-up plan, staff were encouraged to contact their counterparts in other schemes.

They found that a home loans organizer talking to her opposite number, a GP to a GP, produced rich and relevant details which contributed more to long-term commitment than managers' eagerness for 'innovation'. They also recognized that new projects are often in danger of being oversold by those immersed in their development and commissioned an independent evaluation.[6]

The principle aim of the South Derbyshire scheme – good patient outcomes – is echoed in the work of KITTZ, the Institute for Quality and Applied Home Care Innovation in the Netherlands. Its director, Dr Egbert Bosma, emphasized their underlying belief that most people, most of the time, want to be able to function independently in their own homes, even when ill. KITTZ pioneers new ways of making this possible through the safe transfer of hospital-based treatment to the home. Asked about the limits to what patients and family members are willing and safely able to do, he replies 'More than you think.'

The Dutch health system has long had a purchaser/provider split with numerous purchasers in the shape of sick funds, private insurers and municipalities, and providers in the shape of GPs, independent home care organizations and independent hospital organizations. The system is highly regulated and although cost-containment is on the agenda, there is not yet the same imperative as there is in the UK.

There is a strong tradition of home nursing in the Netherlands based on Green Cross Associations. KITTZ has grown out of one of these to become a national development agency focusing on home care programmes. Its bias is twofold: solving the practical problems of providing health care in people's homes, and exploiting technological developments. KITTZ works through a series of home care innovation projects which are documented in the form of protocols, standards, training packages, expert care systems, and then tested and costed in practice. They set out to answer questions such as: Is this method applicable at home? Can this equipment be used at home? Can people work with these instructions? Its goals are to:

• increase people's independence

- increase the possibilities for treatment and nursing at home

- improve the quality of home care by ensuring that everyone concerned has the right information, skills, knowledge and equipment.

Agencies working at the development end of R & D are few and far between and the KITTZ contribution is stimulating, not only because it is rooted in the local experience of a community-based nursing organization, but its approach is practical and the issues being tackled are of international relevance.

Hospital-at-home

Liz Haggard

The interest in hospital-at-home stems from the much discussed shift in the balance of health care from the secondary to the primary and community sector.[1,7,8] The reasons for this shift may be based on political and financial considerations, a positive ideology of maintaining people in their own communities, a wish to minimize the negative experience of institutionalization, or they may express people's wishes to remain in their own homes wherever possible.

This expressed aim of shifting the balance of health care is a feature of care systems in all health and social systems in the West and a key World Health Organization principle. The aim is supported by technological and pharmacological changes which have now made it possible to deliver 'hospital' care in the home. As equipment becomes miniaturized and judgements previously made by experienced and highly trained staff can be captured and computerized, it becomes increasingly possible to create a virtual hospital in the home. Other technological advances, particularly in communications, mean that staff working in the patient's home can be in constant contact with hospital expertise. Finally, there has been a general increase in the quality of accommodation and facilities in the majority of homes so that adequate heating, constant hot water and reasonable bathroom and toilet accommodation are much more the norm than they have ever been.

The experience of being in hospital is no longer culturally regarded as therapeutic in itself; for most people conditions in hospital such as sleep, food, recreation, social contacts and comfort, are less good on a number of measures than conditions in their own home. Hospitals continue to be valued because patients and relatives feel that there will be skilled and constant supervision and safety in the hospital setting and that treatments will be given which will have a benefit for the patient. If hospital-at-home services can offer these two key aspects of a sense of safety and supervision and evidence that skilled treatments can be carried out without the negative aspects of a hospital stay, hospital-at-home may come in time to be the preferred method of treatment for patients. However, the cultural dominance of the hospital model is deeply rooted in the development of health services in this century. We know that these attitudes can be changed – the preferred location for childbirth is an example where we have seen the majority accepting home births at the beginning of the century, moving to hospital births in the post-war period and possibly now moving back to home births as an ideal.

Hospital-at-home is a term with many meanings. For the purposes of this chapter it is defined as a range of services delivered in the patient's home, without which the patient would remain in hospital. It is in every way an alternative to a stay in hospital and is available as a choice for patient, carer, doctor and professional staff caring at home. It is an intensive service delivered to patients who are still in the acute phase of care but who do not require the costly, non-transportable technology which can only be economically provided in a hospital.

Assumptions

Hospital-at-home as a viable model of care is based on a number of assumptions. It assumes that hospital-at-home makes better use of resources in some cases; in particular, it ensures that the scarcest and most costly human and technical resources are concentrated in hospitals and that they are used only when there is no alternative. The model also assumes that it is beneficial to minimize the period away from the person's own home and community and, in particular, that the shorter the stay, the less likely the decay of existing support networks which enabled the patient to live at home before hospitalization. It assumes that rehabilitation will be more effective if it is carried out in the patient's own environment, where the patient has long familiarity and expertise with the environment and the equipment, and has strong motivation to regain their preferred earlier level of functioning. It also assumes that appropriately trained health professionals already work in the community and are available to offer appropriate support to patients in their own homes, and learn additional skills where necessary. Hospital-at-home also assumes to some extent that hospital care has non-benefits which are not found when care is given at home. Examples would be lack of control over the daily timetable, noise and disturbance particularly at night, lack of choice and non-availability of preferred meals and beverages, less one-to-one attention than might be hoped for and assumed, lack of privacy and personalized care routines, a potentially confusingly large number of staff encountered within a 24-hour period and anxiety about conditions at home.

The term *hospital-at-home* in Britain originates with the Peterborough scheme, and although the term has some contradictions, it is helpful in keeping in mind that a hospital-at-home scheme has limited capacity in the same way that a hospital ward does. Those who run hospital-at-home schemes are usually aware of the dangers inherent in pressure to over-expand, causing the scheme to fail because resources are spread too thinly; they tend to describe their schemes as having a limited number of 'beds'. In practice there is greater flexibility than where actual hospital beds are the limiting factor, but the discipline and rigour of thinking in this way is valuable.

Reasons for slow growth

Given the evidence that hospital-at-home is successful on a number of measures,[9,10,11] the main question is why it has been so slow to develop. Although there are now a number of schemes nationally, there are still remarkably few. As stated, culturally there has been a strengthening of the 'hospital is good' model, particularly in the post-war years. The growth in the number of hospitals, with the emphasis in the training of all health professionals on hospital experience rather than community and primary care experience, means that there are a range of resistances to the concept of hospital-at-home. Many of these have been based on a genuinely held belief that patients cannot manage at home, but now that evidence is available other resistances to change in general are probably important factors.

If hospital-at-home were to become widespread, there would be a major change in the pattern of work in hospitals: patients would only be hospitalized in the acute phase for a short time; the rewarding recovery phase would be lost from the hospital staff experience. The recovery phase is rewarding because it shows that treatment has been successful, gives time for a relationship with the patient to develop, and also means that some patients are less dependent than others at any given time with positive effects on stress and workload. If hospital staff have both the acute and recovery phase, there is also more time to carry out arrangements for discharge; the shorter the stay the more rigorous these arrangements have to be.

There are other disincentives for hospitals. Under the current system where purchasers contract with hospital providers to carry out a given level of funded work, there is no incentive for hospitals to reduce that level of work, so the initiative for hospital-at-home might have to come from purchasers. However, the marginal savings from small bed reductions which are the norm in the pilot hospital-at-home developments make almost no difference to the average patient cost for the provider and therefore have no cost benefits for the purchaser either. If the development of a hospital-at-home scheme can enable a ward or a whole section of a hospital to be closed there will be greater cost benefits, but these will still be dwarfed by the general overheads of having a hospital infrastructure.

The greatest savings for purchasers will probably therefore come from using hospital-at-home schemes instead of building hospitals at all. Traditionally we have not been skilled at highlighting savings made by *not* building; a new form of accounting thinking may be needed if progress is to be made to highlight the value of low entry-cost schemes like hospital-at-home. Traditional costing shows that hospital-at-home schemes do not save large sums of money on a cost-per-case basis compared with the costs of the post-acute stage in existing hospitals.[1,12] If costed against the money released by hospitals ceasing to exist or not coming into existence, and the increased ability to respond to change if resources are not tied up in buildings, hospital-at-home would be cost-effective.

Start-up issues

In starting up a hospital-at-home scheme, all the usual problems of project management and change management arise. Project planning has to be meticulous and many schemes underestimate the costs of the infrastructure, such as equipment for the home and communications, necessary to deliver a successful result. The concept of costs such as start-up and launch costs is less well understood in the public sector than in the private sector. Schemes may fail because the purchaser equates good purchasing with driving down costs rather than achieving a successful outcome, so there may be a temptation to underestimate costs.

The need to ensure that a very large number of key players support the scheme requires skilled leadership and change management. Often those responsible for setting up a hospital-at-home scheme have high skills and enthusiasm for service delivery but less skill and less awareness of the need for high level influencing and negotiating skills. Experienced support at this level during the early stages of the setting-up process is often not available and without it there is greater stress and more set-backs. Resistance may be poorly managed, leading to failure or limited success.

Project management and the change management process are particularly complex in a hospital-at-home scheme because hospital consultants and nurses, local general practitioners, community health services staff, social services, and patients' representatives must *all* support the scheme. Failure to gain support from any one of these groups will lead to difficulties and possibly to failure. Failure can result from over-enthusiastic support leading to unrealistic expectations as much as from actual resistance, so the clarity with which the proposals are outlined and constantly restated is also important.

South Derbyshire: learning from experience

South Derbyshire's hospital-at-home scheme is similar to many other schemes, and the key issues have been summarized in a number of articles and working papers.[5,13] One of the objectives in documenting the early stages was to capture information about the processes in the development of the scheme so that others thinking of starting schemes would have detailed guidance and learn from previous mistakes made. Consultancy support has been offered to others setting up schemes and in all cases this emphasis on the process, how support was developed and resistance overcome, was highly valued. Experience shows that without more attention to this aspect of implementing new schemes their replication elsewhere will continue to be patchy and painful.

Key features

- A chief executive was highly involved and a visible champion of the scheme.

- A specific proportion of the budget was set aside for start-up and launch costs, which in later years was available for service delivery.

- A specific budget was allocated to learning from experience elsewhere, in the form of consultancy support and funded visits for staff and clinicians.

- An emphasis on encouraging staff to express their reservations and negative feelings about the scheme rather than 'pushing' the scheme as a good idea.

- A scheme which was clearly nurse-led – the majority of care to patients in hospitals is given by nurses and this is even more true for care in hospital-at-home (the evaluation showed no additional workload for the GPs of hospital-at-home patients).

- A funded, highly-structured training programme including sessions in hospital for professional staff involved in the scheme: maintaining professional standards and confidence is essential. A decision was made to restrict the initial scheme to a particular condition so that training could relate to that condition.

- A decision not to recruit new staff for the hospital-at-home scheme but instead to use existing staff and to recruit staff to replace their time working with current community patients.

- A decision to train hospital-at-home auxiliary staff as generic rehabilitation workers, with a training programme designed by occupational therapy and physiotherapy staff.

- A funded evaluation of the project.

- Public events to launch the hospital-at-home scheme and conferences at planned intervals during the first year, to give non-negotiable deadlines.

- An agreed policy to accept occasional failure and a strategy for dealing with it. Hospital consultants made a commitment to re-admit any hospital-at-home patient if necessary.

- A planned communication strategy to keep a wide range of people informed, a smaller number involved at the commitment level and a very small number working as the operational team taking action.

- Rigorous costing and a commitment to ongoing costing of each case.

It was learned that an excellent home loan service (which had been built up for some years before the hospital-at-home scheme was started) is essential and that transport arrangements have to be fail-safe – sometimes hard to achieve. It was learned that there are hardly any emergencies or re-admissions although everyone raised this prospect as a reservation before the scheme started. It was learned that GPs are confident in their attached district nursing staff and willing to delegate the care of hospital-at-home patients to them; that the staff enjoyed using their acute level skills; that the emphasis on managing a costed package was well accepted and assisted in the good use of appropriate skills; and it was learned again and again that delivering acute level care in the community is a challenge which staff meet successfully if they have good training and infrastructure support in a well managed scheme.

Many lessons were learned about hospital-at-home, but the most important one was that for a significant number of patients, hospital-at-home is a positive alternative to remaining in hospital. Patients who chose it did not regret their decision, in fact they positively valued it. Outcomes were good on all the measures set and hospital-at-home was at least as effective as acute hospital care.

Carer and patient experience

It was learned that from the patients' point of view, it was important to analyse which conditions contributed most to giving the same level of confidence in care at home as they have about hospital care. Guaranteeing patients 24-hour care until they no longer felt they needed it was crucial. So was providing a 'greeting service'; a member of staff at their home to greet them and stay with them on their return from hospital. Patients gained great confidence from having a small number of 'their own' staff and were always able to ask for staff to visit and stay with them – a mobile phone was provided for patients who did not have their own phone.

One criticism of hospital-at-home schemes is that they shift the burden to the carer. There is of course a considerable burden for carers when the patient is in hospital: travel time, cost, loss of ability to care, anxiety, keeping relatives informed. Many hospital-at-home patients in the Southern Derbyshire scheme in fact lived alone, but an essential part of the scheme is that any main carer must agree to hospital-at home admission. Carer satisfaction in the scheme was high.

The future

Since the scheme was started the world has changed and new factors have to be considered. Schemes like hospital-at-home are difficult to deliver for small populations and with the growth of GP fundholding, schemes may need to be re-thought. Health authorities could decide to treat hospital-at-home as a core service not to be included in the calculation of general practitioner funds, but that has non-benefits – it gives GP fundholders no incentive to understand, use and improve hospital-at-home-type schemes and may make the schemes complacent. GP fundholders could buy hospital-at-home schemes and use them as levers to reduce lengths of stay and costs in acute care, and for some very large consortia this might be possible. Starting up hospital-at-home schemes is likely to require central funding initially, but as GP fundholding grows, there will be pressure to release centrally-held funded schemes so that general practitioners can make their own decisions about how to spend on their patients' behalf. If GP fundholders were given funds to purchase acute care and hospital-at-home, they would probably not want to negotiate with two separate providers and would look for a managed acute/hospital-at-home service. However, total purchasing GPs have a greater incentive to develop hospital-at-home schemes because their budgets include all services, not just elective admissions. The acute sector may become interested in providing hospital-at-home, but it lacks the network of trusted and skilled community nursing staff to whom the GP can confidently delegate. As we have seen above there is often no direct incentive for the acute sector in successful hospital-at-home schemes.

Purchaser support for services which change the pattern of care is essential. Hospital-at-home is only one example of innovative patterns of care which will need special protection within a purchaser/provider system. Introducing research-based effective innovations will need protected funding but there will be resistance to top slicing for such funding: there will probably have to be a tapering arrangement. On the provider side, in an increasingly complex and competitive mixed economy of care, where many of the stakeholders feel pressured by the pace of change, it may become harder to secure

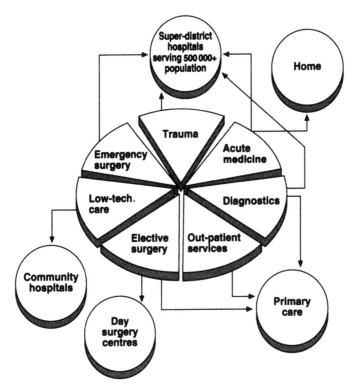

Figure 5.1: Fragmentation of the District General Hospital.

commitment from other providers for schemes like hospital-at-home where the time costs of collaboration can be high.

The search for incentives for all the partners involved in a scheme like hospital-at-home is complex, but without incentives for all players, the scheme will fail. For example, in this hospital-at-home scheme, the incentive for social services was a guarantee that they would not be asked for input until the pre-hospital-at-home day of discharge. This meant that they had no extra services to provide and in many senses benefited because the patient was already well established in their own home by the time social services were provided.

Hospital-at-home schemes are only one part of a mosaic of options which need to be available in a way which is accessible and acceptable to the key decision-makers – general practitioners and consultants – when they plan patient care. The provision of such schemes is one part of the services needed if more care is to be delivered in the primary/community setting.

As Figure 5.1 shows, services once provided only in district general hospitals are moving either to more centralized services or to local primary care.[14] Hospital-at-home schemes are now available for some complex acute conditions, and the range of possibilities is steadily expanding.[9]

Box 5.1: Conditions suitable for hospital-at-home

- Cerebrovascular accidents (CVAs)
- Congestive cardiac failure
- Kidney infections
- Forty-eight hour postoperative hysterectomies
- Cholecystectomies
- Nephrectomies
- Early discharge hip replacements, three days after operation
- Respite care
- Kidney dialysis on a four-year-old
- Terminal care
- HIV and AIDS related illness
- Chemotherapy
- Fractures needing skin traction

Increasing the amount and range of acute care provided outside the acute hospital has many implications for staff in hospital, primary care and community settings. It is important to encourage a wide range of services and not over-invest in one model. Some services should have the key features of hospital-at-home schemes. All should be flexible enough to adjust to the multiple changes which the levers of the NHS reforms, the Community Care Legislation Act and fundholding have added to those of demography, technology and professional and patient aspirations.

Home care innovation: a development agency approach

Egbert Bosma

The Institute for Quality and Applied Home-Care Innovation, (KITTZ) is a young, independent foundation in the Netherlands, financing its activities on a non-profit basis. It was able to start with a one-off subsidy from a regional development fund. The organization originates from the Provincial Green Cross Association in Groningen, in the north of the Netherlands. Green Cross Associations are private organizations which came into being around the turn of the century. Their aim was to control contagious diseases, to improve the population's health in general, and to offer nursing and caring at home. Over the years a network was developed, covering all of the Netherlands. In every city or village, however small, it provides nursing and caring at home, parent and child care, maternity care, information on nutrition and other health promotion activities. Together with general practitioners these organizations offer a unique and firm basis for home care.

Why was a separate organization established for innovation in home care?

New knowledge, equipment and techniques have grown rapidly in the last decade making it not only possible to do more at home but also to do it better. However, existing organizations are cautious about employing new techniques and do so only on a limited scale. KITTZ was founded to bridge the gap between the growing possibilities and everyday practice. KITTZ has its roots in the home care organization, but is not a part of it. It employs a multidisciplinary team of 16 people: nurses, doctors specialized in public health, an engineer, business administrator, public relations officer, programmer and administrative support. KITTZ develops and carries out projects all over the Netherlands and investigates ways in which its methods can be applied elsewhere in Europe.

Why does it put a lot of energy into reinforcing home care?

The main reason is that for most people it is important to function independently in their own homes, even when they are ill, or when things fail to go smoothly due to old age or disability. When asked, 80–90% of people prefer being treated, nursed and taken care of at home, or to die at home. They are prepared to make great efforts to stay at home as long as possible. To have control over one's own life is important for the quality of that life.

Furthermore, the possibilities for home care are extending rapidly. Better living conditions contribute to this; and much of the equipment is getting smaller, safer and easier to operate, so that it can be safely applied outside the hospital.

Another important factor is that cure and care at home are often associated with reduced costs. Experience shows that with many forms of home treatment less professional care is required and the hospital infrastructure is used less. However, the pressure on doctors and nurses working in home care is growing.

What does KITTZ do?

KITTZ works in two fields. The first is about self-help and independence, making sure people have the opportunity to take care of themselves and are no more dependent on the help of family, friends, or professional carers than is strictly necessary. It is concerned with aids to independent living, good equipment and furniture, and adaptations to the home. The second is nursing and treatment at home, the field of home care and hospital-at-home.

As a development agency KITTZ's activities are geared to innovation, implementation and quality improvement. By innovation we mean process innovation, developing so-called new care processes, for example, when treatment is moved from the hospital to the home. Product innovation plays a less important role. Innovations, however, only make sense when they are actually applied. Therefore KITTZ's activities are strongly focused on implementation; the application of techniques in practice. This means supporting and guiding care providers and their organizations in applying new methods. One of the essentials for implementation on a large scale is the development and recording of a methodology, making it possible to pass on knowledge and expertise. It puts a lot of energy and time into developing these materials. KITTZ's third group of activities is focused on quality improvement; not only the quality of the care processes, but the skills and expertise of those who undertake them.

Examples of KITTZ programmes

1 Infusion-therapy at home
  Cancer pain treatment
  IV administration of antibiotics
  Tube feeding
  Chemotherapy
  Total parenteral feeding

2 Respiratory disorders at home
  Health effects of reduction of mites in house dust
  Treatment of congenital alveolar dysplasia (respiratory
    distress syndrome of newborn)
  Home care for patients with severe emphysema
  Expert system on sanitation of houses of patients with
    allergic asthma

3 Cystic fibrosis home care
  IV administration of antibiotics
  Tube feeding
  Liquid oxygen

4 Wound care and wound treatment
  Development of an expert system
  Tube feeding and pressure sores (decubitus ulcers)
  Effectiveness of materials for prevention of pressure sores
  Diabetic foot

5 Traction therapy at home
  Traction therapy with infants and adults

6 Housing and self-support
Demonstration house 'Zuidhorn'
User experience of equipment
Home care technology for the elderly

As an independent development agency KITTZ is not a
provider organization in competition with others. It works for
hospitals, home care organizations, purchasers of health
services and the government – in short, for everyone who is
convinced of the importance of increasing the possibilities for
home care. Many different agencies make use of the outcome of
its work. In order to achieve this, it was necessary to develop a
methodology that could be applied in various situations. When
developing a new care process for the home, the starting point
is always the patient and the problems he/she encounters. The
solution is based on this. The elements that are of crucial
importance are systematically analysed and laid down. Then,
from experience, the expertise and skills necessary to carry out
treatment at home are mapped, along with what equipment
can be used, how it should be used, which demands the
provider organization must comply with, and the costs and
financial implications. Thorough information is of the utmost
importance, not only for successful treatment but also for conveying project results. Basically, the stages in the process and
the problems patients experience are comparable throughout
Western Europe. Organizational structures and financial mechanisms are unique in each country, but the heart of the matter,
the treatment process, is by and large the same. KITTZ's
methodology makes it possible to adapt the care process to regional variations, without detracting from its safety or quality.
   Another critical factor to the way it works is to create an
expert network from around the country to participate in the
planning and implementing of each project. At present it is
engaged in 21 innovation projects in several different fields.
Two goals are realized through this network. First, the necessary expertise from doctors, chemists, nurses, representatives of
patients, research institutes, companies etc., is mobilized to develop high quality projects and excellent products. Second, a
roll-out programme is created outside the experimental zone, to
test the implementation of the results elsewhere in the country.

KITTZ's innovation projects are formed in actual practice. After the initial development stage the new care process is put into practice and modified on the basis of patients' daily experience making use of regular care provision. When necessary, the nurses give additional specialist help. They ensure that all information is gathered and processed into protocols, which in the end contribute to a home-care programme. A KITTZ home-care programme is the key to conveying project results. It is a structured and standardized description of the care process at home. It not only describes what must be done, but also how it should be done. This method also enables KITTZ to withdraw when the project is finished and allow the new treatment process to continue without it. It works as a catalyst. By remaining neutral in the entire innovation flow it can bring parties together to work in new ways who would otherwise fail to reach fruitful cooperation.

Occasionally there are negative aspects for the staff working this way. During a project they often become a recognized authority on treatment, with all the benefits this brings, such as expert status and invitations to conferences. When the project is finished, however, they must withdraw and work their way into a new project. This keeps things alive and fascinating, but taking leave of success is not always easy. KITTZ looks for ways to maintain some staff involvement in a subject in order to maintain the expertise which has been built-up and to make sure that the home-care programme remains up to date.

Summary

KITTZ is an organization with its roots in community-based health services. It works as an independent agency to create more and better opportunities for independent living and for care and treatment at home. It was formed to bridge the gap between everyday practice and the growing possibilities of new ways of providing services out of hospitals. The starting point for each development project is the experience of patients and the methodology is designed to ensure practical applicability and a roll-out programme beyond the innovation stage.

References

Chapter 1

1 EL(94)79. (1994) *Developing NHS purchasing and GP fund-holding: towards a primary care-led NHS.* Department of Health, Leeds.

2 Taylor D. (1991) *Developing primary care. Opportunities for the 1990s.* Research Report 10, King's Fund, London.

3 Haggard L. (1990) A safety net for mending. *Health Service Journal,* **100**:5223.

4 Titmuss RM. (1963) *Essays on the Welfare State.* Unwin University Books, London.

5 Balint M. (1957) *The doctor, his patient, and the illness.* Pitman Medical, London.

6 RCGP Working Party. (1972) The future general practitioner. Learning and teaching. *British Medical Journal,* for RCGP, London.

7 Pratt J. (1995) *Practitioners and Practices: a conflict of values?* Radcliffe Medical Press, Oxford.

8 Plamping D. (1995) *From general practice to primary care organisation.* Unpublished working paper, King's Fund, London.

9 Moore GT. (1992) The disappearing generalist. *Milbank Quarterly,* **70(2)**:361–79.

10 Allsop J. (1990) *Changing primary care: The role of facilitators.* King's Fund, London.

11 London Health Planning Consortium. (1981) *Primary Health Care in Inner London. Report of a studygroup.* (Chairman: ED Acheson). DHSS, London.

12 Hughes J and Gordon P. (1992) *An optimal balance? Primary health care and acute hospital services in London.* London Initiative Working Paper no. 8, King's Fund, London.

13 Dept. of Health. (1989) *General practice in the National Health Service. A new contract.* HMSO, London.

14 Gillam S *et al.* (1994) *Community Oriented Primary Care.* King's Fund, London.

15 Plamping D. (1995) *Putting primary care centre stage.* NHS Handbook 10th Edition. NAHAT, Birmingham. 27–31.

16 Beardshaw V and Robinson R. (1990) *New for Old? Prospects for nursing in the 1990s.* Research Report 8, King's Fund, London.

17 Patients First. (1979) *Consultative paper on the structure and management of the National Health Service in England and Wales.* HMSO, London.

18 Dalley G. (1989) Community health services today. In: Hughes J (ed) *The future of community health services.* King's Fund, London.

19 Dept. of Health and Social Security. (1986) *Neighbourhood nursing – a focus for care. Report of the Community Nursing Review Team.* (Chairman: Mrs Julia Cumberlege). HMSO, London.

20 Welsh Office. (1988) *Nursing in the community – a team approach for Wales. Report of the Review of Community Nursing in Wales.* (Chairman: Mrs Noreen Edwards). Welsh Office, Cardiff.

21 Cornwell J. (1989) *The Consumers' View: Elderly People and Community Health Services.* King's Fund, London.

22 Kalsi N and Constantinides P. (1989) *Working towards racial equality in health care: the Haringey experience.* King's Fund, London.

23 Brown P and Gordon P. (1987) *Cumberlege in Action.* King's Fund, London.

24 Brown P, Gordon P and Hughes J. (1988) *Changing School Health Services.* King's Fund, London.

25 Dalley G, Hughes J and King C. (1987) *Decentralising community health services.* King's Fund, London.

26 Hughes J. (ed) (1990) *Enhancing the quality of community nursing.* King's Fund, London.

27 Winn KE and Quick A. (1990) *User Friendly Services. Guidelines for managers of community health services.* King's Fund, London.

28 Working for Patients. (1989) HMSO, London. Cmnd 555.

29 Griffiths R. (1988) *Community Care: an agenda for action. A report to the Secretary of State for Social Services.* HMSO, London.

30 Hughes J. (ed) (1989) *The future of community health services.* King's Fund, London.

31 Constantinides P and Gordon P. (1990) A model of service. *Health Service Journal,* **100:**5222.

32 Audit Commission. (1992) *Homeward Bound: A New Course for Community Health.* HMSO, London.

33 Roy S. (1990) *Nursing in the Community.* A report of the Working Group, North West Thames Regional Health Authority, London.

34 Haggard E. (1993) Integrating primary and secondary care. In: Cook H and Garside P (eds) *Managing NHS Trusts*. Longman, Harlow.

35 Plamping D. (1995) Solutions – but for which problems? In: Anand P and McGuire A (eds) *Current Issues in the NHS: Implementing the Health Care Reforms*. Stephen Rutt and Macmillan, London.

36 Neuburger J. (1992) London after Tomlinson: Community Health Services. *British Medical Journal*, **305**:1486–8.

37 Ellis N. (1994) *Community Health Services: Health News Briefing*. Association of Community Health Councils of England and Wales, London.

38 Bunce C. (1993) Hospital at Home is a feasible option. *Fundholding*, 7 October, 14–16.

39 Office for Public Management. (1995) *Beyond the Looking Glass. The future for community trusts*. Office for Public Management, London.

40 Benjamin AE. (1993) An historical perspective on home care policy. *Milbank Quarterly*, **71**(1):129–65.

41 Huntington J. (1995) *Managing the practice: whose business?* Radcliffe Medical Press, Oxford.

42 Meads G. (ed) (1995) *Future Options for General Practice*. Radcliffe Medical Press, Oxford.

Chapter 2

1 Hughes J and Gordon P. (1993) *Hospitals and primary care*. King's Fund, London.

2 Audit Commission. (1986) *Making a Reality of Community Care*. HMSO, London.

3 Wilkin D and Dornan C. (1990) *General practitioner referrals to hospital. A review of research and its implications for policy and practice.* Centre for Primary Care Research, Dept. of General Practice, University of Manchester.

4 Marks L. (1994) *Seamless Care or Patchwork Quilt? Discharging patients from acute hospital care.* Research report 17. King's Fund, London.

5 Hunter D. (1990) 'Managing the cracks': Management development for health care interfaces. *International Journal of Health Planning and Management,* **5**:7–14.

6 Schon D. (1971) *Beyond the Stable State.* Temple Smith, London.

7 Johnson G and Scholes K. (1988) *Exploring Corporate Strategy.* Prentice Hall, London.

8 McMullen T. (1993) *Facilitation of Change in a Primary Health Care Environment.* Project report for Dip. Man. Studies, Sheffield.

9 Balint M. (1957) *The doctor, his patient, and the illness.* Pitman Medical, London.

10 Axelrod R. (1990) *The evolution of co-operation.* Penguin, London.

11 Ellis N. (1994) *Community Health Services. Health News Briefing.* Association of Community Health Councils for England and Wales. London.

12 Office for Public Management. (1995) *Beyond the Looking Glass. The Future of Community NHS Trusts.* Office for Public Management, London.

13 Allsop J. (1990) *Changing primary care: The role of facilitators.* King's Fund, London.

14 Standing Committee on Postgraduate Medical and Dental Education. (1994) *The Health of the Nation: Implications for postgraduate and continuing medical and dental education.* SCOPME, London.

15 Boufford J. (1994) *Shifting the balance from acute to community health care.* King's Fund, London.

16 Rogers M. (1993) The growing pains of community child health. *Archives of Disease in Childhood,* **68**:140–3.

17 British Paediatric Association. (1993) Towards a Combined Child Health Service. BPA, London.

18 British Paediatric Association. (1992) Management models in established, combined or integrated child health services. BPA, London.

Chapter 3

1 Glendinning C, Bailey J, Jones J *et al.* (1995) *Primary Care Resource Centres in England: an initial survey.* National Primary Care Research and Development Centre, Manchester.

Chapter 5

1 Marks L. (1991) *Home and hospital care: redrawing the boundaries.* Research Report 9, King's Fund, London.

2 Hughes J and Gordon P. (1993) *Hospitals and primary care.* King's Fund, London.

3 Gaze H. (1989) Learning to COPE. *Nursing Times,* **85**(26), 16–17.

4 Smits A, Mansfield S and Singh S. (1990) Facilitating care of patients with HIV infection by hospital and primary care teams. *British Medical Journal,* **300**:241–3.

5 Haggard L and Benjamin B. (1992) All Systems Go. *Health Service Journal,* **102**:5313.

6   O'Cathain A. (1991) *An evaluation of the South Derbyshire Hospital at Home Scheme*. Southern Derbyshire Health Authority, Derby.

7   Stocking B. (1992) Moving acute health care into the home. In: Costain D and Warner M (eds) *From Hospital to Home Care: the potential for acute service provision in the home*. King's Fund, London.

8   Boufford J. (1994) *Shifting the balance from acute to community health care*. King's Fund, London.

9   Bunce C. (1993) Hospital at Home is a feasible option. *Fundholding*, **2**(18):14–6.

10   Hackman B. (1993) There's no place like home: early discharge after hysterectomy. *Nursing Times*, **89**:28.

11   Taylor J, Goodman M and Luesley D. (1993) Is home best? Early discharge effects on patients after hysterectomy. *Nursing Times*, **89**:31.

12   Hollingsworth W, Todd C, Parker M *et al.* (1993) Cost analysis of early discharge after hip fracture. *British Medical Journal*, **307**:903–6.

13   Southern Derbyshire Community Health Services Trust. (1990) *Three reports on Hospital at Home: Getting started; Three months on; Evaluation*. Southern Derbyshire Community Health Services Trust, Derby.

14   Laing W. (1994) *Managing the NHS: past, present and agenda for the future*. Office of Health Economics, London.

Index

Page references in italics indicate tables and figures. In some cases there may also be textual references on these pages.

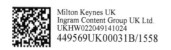